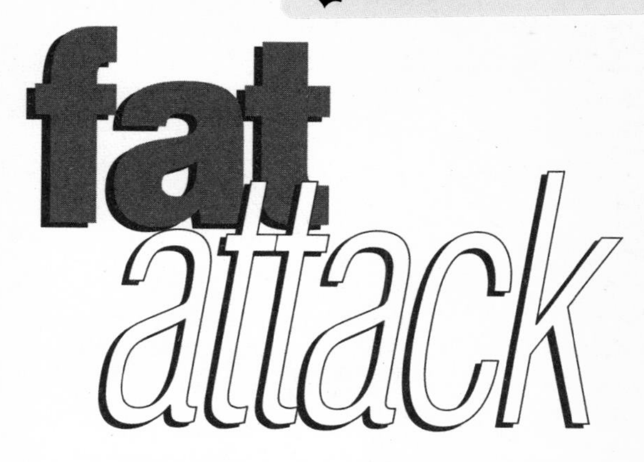

The no-hunger way to a fitter, leaner body and a healthy heart

Judith Wills

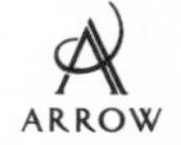

Also in Vermilion by Judith Wills

SIZE 12 IN 21 DAYS
COMPLETE SPEED SLIMMING SYSTEM
SLIM FOR LIFE

First published in 1995
1 3 5 7 9 10 8 6 4 2

First published in the United Kingdom in 1995
by Vermilion Arrow
an imprint of Ebury Press
Random House, 20 Vauxhall Bridge Road,
London SW1V 2SA

Random House Australia (Pty) Limited
20 Alfred Street, Milsons Point, Sydney,
New South Wales 2061, Australia

Random House New Zealand Limited
18 Poland Road, Glenfield,
Auckland 10, New Zealand

Random House South Africa (Pty) Limited
PO Box 337, Bergvlei, South Africa

Random House UK Limited Reg. No. 954009

ISBN 0 09 949761 1

Designed by Roger Walker
Photography by Jon Stewart

Printed in Great Britain by
Cox & Wyman Ltd, Reading

Contents

Acknowledgements

With special thanks to:
Miranda Llewellyn for helping so much with the toning exercise programme in chapter 6 and checking for safety; Lisa Brockwell for demonstrating the exercises. Thanks also to Jan Bowmer, Niccy Cowen, Sarah Bennie, Roger Walker, Tony Allen and Jane Turnbull for all their help along the way.

Introduction

You know the scene. Every now and then you decide it's time to lose a bit of weight; cut out chocolate and chips; start a fitness regime; get healthier. But somehow it never lasts, does it? Sooner or later, everything's back as it was. Except, with every year, is it your imagination, or are you a bit fatter; a bit more unfit, and a bit more entrenched in the habits keeping you that way?

Most of us know that it's a good idea to cut down on the fat in our diets and to avoid *getting* fat. For over a decade, the Department of Health (DoH) and the World Health Organisation (WHO) have been urging us to reduce our fat intake. Not only does eating too much fat keep your body fat, but it has also been conclusively shown that a diet high in saturated fats can *double* your risk of heart disease. By swopping to the right type of reduced-fat diet you can not only lose weight painlessly, but actually cut your risk of heart disease by up to a half!

With facts like these available, isn't it *astounding* that, as a nation, we in Britain are *still* eating as much fat as we ever were? *Over 40 per cent of the food we eat is pure fat.*

WHY?

Well, according to my own research and a recent nationwide survey, the answer is quite simple. We like our food – and dislike change – too much to make what we see as difficult and unpalatable alterations in our diets.

We want to be slim, we want to be healthy – but not if it is at the expense of our enjoyment of our food, takes longer, or costs more.

Well – if that sounds like you, my message to you is this:

You don't HAVE *to make drastic changes to your diet in order to cut your fat down to levels that can get and keep you lean and protect your heart.* You don't have to be bored or deprived or hungry. *You don't have to be a martyr to the cause.*

You can 'attack the fat' – both in your food and on your body – and do your heart a favour too, while eating a tasty, delicious diet that includes all the types of food you've come to love so much ... curries, roasts, Chinese, Italian, Mexican, desserts, treats. You can eat *all* these and *still* keep your fat intake to well within official guidelines.

And this is the book that shows you how.

I wrote *Fat Attack* because I am fed up with low-fat diets and books that make it all seem like a pain and a misery. I wrote it because I am fed up with undoing the damage that unnecessarily tough, extreme dietary advice has done. The kind of advice that restricts, and forbids too much, puts off more people than it helps and encourages us to say, 'Forget the diet – I'm going to eat when I like and stay fat!'

Now it's time to set the record straight. I hope you will read *Fat Attack* and be inspired when you see how well you can eat and how few radical changes you need to make to your diet or your lifestyle.

I've used all the latest research – and my own fifteen years' experience and common sense – to produce a no-fuss, no-hunger plan that is 'real eating' rather than 'being on a diet'. All you need to know for an easy, inexpensive, pleasant reduced-fat diet for the rest of your life is here in this book.

And, lastly, because most of us have the same attitude to exercise as we do to cutting fat ('If it's easy, I'll do it'), I've also produced what I believe is the simplest-*ever* fat-burning exercise programme. It will not only help to get you lean but will also improve your general fitness and, again, help you to a healthy heart, while being suitable for all ages and all fitness levels.

The *Fat Attack* programme is as suitable for men (and the whole family) as it is for women. So please, if you are a woman buying *Fat Attack* – don't keep it to yourself! The eating plan, with very minor adjustments, is ideal for weight maintenance, so even if family members don't need to shed pounds they can still follow it. The *Fat Attack* diet incorporates *all* the latest recommendations on eating for a healthy heart – I've built in *all* the known protective factors, about which you'll learn more in the pages to come.

Please share *Fat Attack* and do your family a favour. This book is for you – and the people you care for.

To Tony

IMPORTANT

If you have a medical condition or are pregnant, the diet and exercises described in this book should not be followed without first consulting your doctor. All guidelines and warnings should be read carefully, and the author and publisher cannot accept responsibility for injuries or damage arising out of a failure to comply with the same.

CHAPTER 1

Fat – The Burning Questions

Before we begin the campaign to reduce the fat in our food – and on our bodies – let's get the fat facts straightened out first.

There is so much conflicting 'evidence' presented by so many different experts and organizations that you are probably now totally confused about fat and its role in our diet, as well as its effect on our weight and our health.

New theories, research and trial results come in from all over the world with alarming regularity – and each report seems to conflict with the one that went before. But all the 'fat facts' in this chapter are based upon the most widely accepted knowledge and recommendations currently available.

The World Health Organisation (WHO), the Department of Health (DoH) and the British Nutrition Foundation have been my major sources of information and data for *Fat Attack*.

As a result, the messages in the book will, I am sure, be clear, strong, positive, simple to understand – and effective.

WHAT IS FAT?

In simple terms, the fat that we eat is mainly made up of different fatty acids bound together with glycerine. What makes, for example, corn oil different from butterfat is largely the different proportions of these fatty acids that each fat contains.

Fat's primary use in our diet is as an energy source. Surplus fat not used for energy is laid down as body fat which can be converted back to energy in the future should the need arise. The other foods in our diet that supply us with energy (calories) are carbohydrates, protein and alcohol.

Dietary fat is not just contained in the obvious fats, such as butter and lard. Oil is fat, too, and many everyday 'high-protein' foods such as milk and eggs, and 'high-carbohydrate' foods such as cakes and biscuits, have a high fat content. Sixty-seven per cent of the calories in an egg, for instance, are fat calories. Even some fruits and vegetables, such as bananas and mushrooms, contain a little fat.

IS ALL FAT BASICALLY THE SAME?

No. There are several different types of dietary fat which can be simply grouped into the following categories:

Saturated fat

This is the kind of fat that is likely to be solid at room temperature and is found mainly in animal products such as meat, lard and dairy produce. The only plant to contain high levels of saturated fat is the coconut.

Unsaturated fat

This is the fat that is likely to be liquid at room temperature and is found in greatest quantity in vegetable oils.

Mono-unsaturated fat is found in largest quantities in olive oil, groundnut (peanut) oil and rapeseed oil.

Poly-unsaturated fat is found in largest quantities in oils which stay liquid at cool temperatures, such as corn oil, sunflower oil, soyabean oil and safflower oil.

There are also special kinds of poly-unsaturated fats called the *long chain n-3 fatty acids*, sometimes known as the 'omega-3s'. These n-3 fatty acids are found almost exclusively in oily fish such as herrings, mackerel and salmon.

Trans fatty acids

These are vegetables or fish oils which have been hardened (hydrogenated) by manufacturers and used in a variety of commercial products such as margarine and baked goods. This hydrogenating process alters the basic composition of the oils so that, as trans fatty acids, they are now thought to have a similar effect in our bodies as saturated fat.

None of the fats or fatty foods are made up of just one of these sorts of fat. Most are a combination. For instance, beef contains only around 50 per cent saturated fat, the remaining 50 per cent being made up of a combination of mono- and poly-unsaturated fats.

Even the oils that most people think of as being poly-unsaturated – e.g. sunflower oil – contain mono- and poly-unsaturates, too.

Butter fat is two-thirds saturated; most of the rest is mono-unsaturated.

HOW MUCH FAT DO WE CURRENTLY EAT IN THE UK?

The average British diet contains around 40 per cent of its calories in the form of fats. (Obviously, then, a lot of people are eating *more* than this.)

The typical man on a normal maintenance diet of about 2,550 calories a day will eat around 113g (4oz) of pure fat a day, 45g – nearly 2oz – of this will be saturated fat.

The typical woman on a maintenance diet of 1,940 calories a day will be eating around 86g (over 3oz) of fat and 35g (over 1oz) of saturated fat a day.

A very overweight person, who is likely to be consuming many more calories than average a day, could easily be eating his or her way through *half a pound* – nearly a quarter of a kilo – of fat a day.

The fact is that in Britain and other countries of the Western world, we eat huge quantities of fat.

HOW MUCH FAT SHOULD WE BE EATING?

The World Health Organisation (WHO), the Department of Health (DoH) and the British Nutrition Foundation recommend that we cut our total fatty acid intake per day to 30 per cent of total calorie intake *as a maximum*. They also recommend that the *proportion* of fats we eat should be approximately:

10 per cent maximum saturated
2 per cent maximum trans fatty acids
12 per cent mono-unsaturated
6 per cent poly-unsaturated.

Because we currently don't eat more than the recommended levels of the mono- and poly-unsaturated fats anyway, we should lower our total fat figure by reducing the amount of *saturated* and *trans* fatty acids that we eat.

In fact, according to the WHO, there is *no* lower limit on the amount of saturated or trans fatty acids we should eat.

For weight maintenance, the 30 per cent total fat intake figure is reasonable. However, research studies on both sides of the Atlantic have found that for people who want to lose weight, a further reduction to bring total fat intake to around 20–25 per cent of total daily calorie intake may make losing weight much easier. (More about that later on.)

BUT WHY, EXACTLY, SHOULD WE EAT LESS FAT?

For the sake of our health – and our weight.

The WHO and the DoH both recommend us to cut our fat intake because the relationship between a high-fat diet – particularly the Western high-*saturated*-fat diet – and all forms of heart and circulatory disease appears to be conclusive.

Coronary heart disease (CHD) is the biggest single cause of death in the UK and many other countries in both men and women. In the UK about two million people have some symptoms of CHD. UK death rates from CHD are some of the highest in the world, and CHD is by far the biggest cause of *premature death* in both men and women.

In February 1994, all the evidence from the largest international studies and trials concerning the relationship between a high-fat diet, blood cholesterol and heart disease was combined and published in the *British Medical Journal*, and the results appear to prove conclusively that lowering our total fat intake to around 27 per cent of total energy intake and lowering our saturated fat intake to around 8 per cent of total energy intake would give a staggering *50 per cent* reduction in deaths from heart disease in people aged 55–64. Even a modest reduction in fat intake to 35 per cent total fat and 13 per cent saturated fat would reduce deaths from heart disease by 50 per cent at age 40, 40 per cent at age 50, 30 per cent at age 60 and 20 per cent at age 70.

And the same report showed that it takes only *two years* of adopting the lower-fat diet for most of the benefit to be felt, and only five years for the full reduction in risk to be achieved.

In other words, if a man aged 35 who currently eats a high-fat/high-saturated-fat diet alters that diet to within the guidelines *now*, he will, by the age of 40, have halved his risk of heart disease.

And this link is not only of interest to men – heart disease in women, especially at a younger age, is growing, too.

Weight problems

Obesity (chronic overweight) is associated with heart disease (the more overweight you are, the more chance you have of developing heart disease). And obesity and overweight are most commonly found in people who eat a high-fat diet.

Obese people are more likely than normal-weight people to suffer from high blood pressure, which itself is a risk factor for both stroke and heart disease.

But obesity is not just linked with heart problems. If you are much overweight, you run an increased risk of developing one or more of the following: *gallstones*, *osteoarthritis*, *mid-life-onset diabetes*, *infertility*, *varicose veins* and *some forms of cancer*.

Eating less fat is not the *only* way you can help your health and your weight, of course. Later on in *Fat Attack* we'll be looking at your diet as a whole and seeing what else we can do to make it healthier.

You should also take enough exercise (which we'll be looking at in chapter 6), give up smoking if you do, and avoid too much stress.

SO WHAT IS IT THAT MAKES FAT SO BAD FOR US?

It is far from true to say that 'fat is bad for you'. We all need some fat in our diets.

There are various reasons for this.

One is that there are two 'essential fatty acids' – linoleic acid and alpha-linolenic acid (both poly-unsaturates) – that our bodies need in small quantities for good health and can only get from food.

Another reason is that three of our most important vitamins – A, D and E – are what is known as 'fat-soluble', and we need to take in some fat so that these vitamins can carry out their vital work.

A third reason is that the latest research indicates that several of the poly-unsaturated fatty acids may protect us against many kinds of disease. For instance, it may be possible to treat osteoporosis (thinning of the bones as we get older) with two fatty acids – GLA and EPA for short.

It is known that the 'long chain n-3' fatty acids found mostly in fish, especially oily fish, when eaten regularly reduce the tendency of the blood to clot and therefore offer protection against circulatory and heart disease. And it has been known for a long time that both poly-unsaturates and mono-unsaturates protect against heart disease by their action in reducing certain types of artery-blocking cholesterol in the blood.

So you see – when it comes to your heart and your health, some fats are positively saintly!

A further reason for including fat in your diet is that a certain amount makes our food palatable. If we didn't eat any fat, many of us would become too thin – and extreme thinness is associated with almost as many physical problems and diseases as is fatness.

Taking all this into account, it's easy to see why it would be foolish to try to adopt a 'fat-free' diet (even if that were possible).

There is even no point in reducing your fat intake to a *very* low level – say, below 20 per cent. That is because, as we've seen, reasonable amounts of the mono- and poly-unsaturated fats in our diets probably offer many more benefits than drawbacks.

No – what we appear to have got wrong in the modern West is that we eat far too much *saturated* fat for good health, and it is these excess quantities of the high-saturated-fat foods, such as full-fat dairy produce, fatty cuts of meat, pastries and baked goods, that we should mostly try to cut down on.

Saturated fat is the only fat for which the WHO has not set recommended lower limits. In other words, if you eat *no* saturated fat, it won't do you any harm and will probably do you a lot of good.

The reason that a lot of saturated fat is not good for us is that a high-saturated-fat diet tends to raise blood cholesterol levels by stimulating the production of 'low density lipoproteins', which often leads to clogging up of arteries so that the blood circulation is affected. Clots in the blood are more easily formed, and these can cause strokes and heart attack.

The latest research also strongly indicates that trans fatty acids may have a similar effect. The basis of the *Fat Attack* diet is to reduce the intake of both saturated and trans fats.

AND WHY DOES A HIGH-FAT DIET MAKE US FAT?

Of course, not everybody who eats a lot of fat gets fat – some people are very active and need a lot of calories to maintain a normal weight. (Nevertheless, if they eat a lot of saturated fat, they are still increasing their risk of heart disease.) Other people have a naturally high metabolic rate (the rate at which we burn off the food we eat for energy) and don't seem to get fat however many chips they eat!

But, as a general rule, it is easy for most of us to put on weight if we eat a lot of fat. There are various reasons for this.

- *If you eat a high-fat diet you are probably eating far more calories than you realize.* Gram for gram, fat contains over twice the calories of carbohydrate, protein or alcohol. Every gram of fat contains 9 calories, so a teaspoonful contains around 45 calories. And because fat is so 'melty', it slips down our throats almost without us noticing. Think of eating five chocolates out of a box (around 200 calories) compared with eight Ryvitas (200 calories) one after the other and you'll see what I mean!

  I could 'hide' four or five hundred calories' worth of fat on your dinner plate so that your meal hardly looked any different from a lower-fat one – and you'd eat it just as quickly and not feel any more full at the end.
- *Your body easily converts surplus fat in your diet (that which isn't needed for energy) into fat on you.* All the latest research shows that the fat in your diet is much more easily converted into body fat than either protein or carbohydrate. That's hardly surprising, really, as carbohydrate and protein both need to undergo radical changes to turn into fat – whereas fat is, well, *already* fat! Research carried out at the part-government-funded Dunn Clinical Nutrition Centre in Cambridge also seems to show that when we eat carbohydrate, protein or alcohol our metabolism apparently responds to the fact that food is being eaten and begins to burn it off straight away. But when we eat fat, the fat seems to slip in unnoticed, and the metabolic rate stays the same. This could be another reason why fat makes us fat.

- *Fat in our Western diet is often combined with sugar in 'binge' foods.* Although some people, certainly, are 'addicted' to cheese, cream, butter and meat, the foods that contribute most to our high-saturated-fat diet are manufactured foods – the cakes, pastries, biscuits, sweets, puddings and so on that are combinations of fat and sugar or fat and flour, or all three. These highly refined foods are the ones many people find hard to resist – partly because of that 'melt in the mouth' fat feeling; and partly because these refined foods tend to cause highs and lows in our blood sugar levels which can make us crave them more (more on that later).
- *High-fat meals don't look like much on the plate – unless we eat much* more *of them.* Think of a tiny party-size pork pie. Put it on your lunch plate and you are likely to put on another, and then add some bread and butter and a few more bits and pieces because that one pork pie doesn't look like enough to feed a kitten. Yet that tiny pie will contain around 300 calories – mostly fat. The same is true of a small piece of full-fat Cheddar cheese. It doesn't look much so we've got to have more. *All* the high-fat high-calorie foods are deceptively small – and encourage us to keep on eating them.

SO, IS A LOW-FAT DIET THE ONLY WAY TO LOSE BODY FAT?

Strictly speaking, no. To lose weight you simply have to take in – in the form of food – fewer calories than you are using up in energy. So if you are using up, say, 2,000 calories a day and you eat a daily diet of 1,000 calories of pure fat, you will still lose weight.

But this would be (a) unhealthy and (b) hard to stick to. Unhealthy because of all the reasons we've discussed and because you would be falling short of all the vital vitamins, minerals, etc. as well as protein and carbohydrate. And hard to follow because, as we've seen, 1,000 calories' worth of high-fat food looks like very little food indeed.

The advantages of losing weight on a diet that restricts fat (particularly saturated fat) but allows you plenty of carbohydrate foods and sufficient protein are not only that this is a generally healthy way to eat, in any event, but also that such a diet, it now seems, allows you to slim without feeling hungry and without counting calories as such. In other words, shed your body fat by eating less fat, and the task of slimming becomes much easier.

Two separate, important controlled trials by well-respected research centres (Cornell University in the USA and the Dunn Clinical Nutrition Centre in the UK) found that people fed a diet with the fat content reduced to 20–25 per cent of total calories, but who were allowed to eat normal quantities of the high-'complex'-carbohydrate foods, such as bread, potatoes, pasta, rice, grains, pulses, fruit and vegetables, lost weight steadily.

In other words, these trials demonstrated that if you keep the fat content of your diet reasonably low, you can literally have as much food on your plate as ever *and* for the most part dispense with calorie-counting – and still lose weight.

This means that anyone who has had problems in trying to stick to a reduced-calorie diet in the past due to hunger or feelings of deprivation or lack of time will find a reduced-fat diet much more pleasant and easy to follow.

These are exactly the principles behind the Fat Attack *diet system.* I've cut the fat – but not the food. With the 30-day *Fat Attack* plan (which is repeatable for as long as you like) you can lose body fat

- *without hunger*
- *without deprivation*
- *without fiddly weighing of most of your foods*
- *without losing pleasure in your eating*
- *and without feeling isolated* (because everyone can enjoy *your* food too).

So, looked at logically, the reduced-fat, high-carbohydrate diet *is* the only sensible way to shed body fat – while doing your health a big favour.

CAN I LOSE BODY FAT THROUGH EXERCISE?

Yes, you can. Just as a reduced-calorie diet produces fat loss by ensuring that your body has to burn up its own fat for energy, so regular exercise of the right type can achieve a similar fat-burning effect – except that it is more immediate because within a few minutes of beginning exercise you are actually burning up your fat stores for fuel!

However, it is hard for most normal, busy people to fit in enough daily exercise to lose more than, at most, half a pound (225g) a week or so of fat through exercise alone. That is because you have to burn up around 3,500 calories' worth of energy to lose one pound (450g) of body fat.

However, even a half a pound a week fat loss through exercise makes a very useful contribution to your fat-loss programme when you look at it over the months. Exercise also has benefits for your heart and body in many other ways (see chapter 6) which is why the *Take Thirty* programme in that chapter is an essential part of your *Fat Attack* plan.

HOW MUCH BODY FAT DO I NEED TO LOSE?

There are two methods that will give you a good, free indication of whether you need to shed body fat. (You can get your body fat percentage tested at a clinic or health club, but that's expensive.)

I say 'indication' because there is no rule about *exactly* how much fat you should carry and certainly no exact point at which one ounce *under* it you are healthy and one ounce *over* it you are not!

Waist to hip ratio

Much research done in the last decade suggests that it is body fat *distribution* that is as important as what you weigh in deciding whether or not you should shed fat. It is now known that *central* fat distribution – i.e., fat around your waist and stomach – poses a greater risk to your health than lower body fat. In other words, the typical, pear-shaped woman has much less to worry about than a pot-bellied, apple-shaped man. Of course, not everyone is an exact pear or an exact apple, and there are plenty of apple-shaped women as well as men.

You can easily work out whether your fat is 'centrally distributed' or not by working out your *waist to hip ratio*.

All you do is divide your waist measurement by your hip measurement and the result is your WHR. For instance, if your waist is 30 inches (75cm) and your hips are 37 inches (93cm) you WHR is 0.81.

The bigger your waist in relation to your hips, the higher the figure will be.

For women, an average WHR is 0.75, and for men, 0.95. Figures below those averages indicate a 'pear shape', ones above indicate an 'apple shape'.

Use this WHR in conjunction with method two that follows and you should have a very good guide as to whether you do need to shed body fat.

Body Mass Index

The Body Mass Index (BMI) is the modern equivalent of the height/weight charts. This is how you work it out:

- Convert your current weight into kilograms. (Say, you are 10 stone 7 lbs – that is (10 × 14 + 7) 147 lbs. Each kg is 2.2 lbs, so divide 147 by 2.2. You are 66.8kg.)
- Convert your height into metres by multiplying your height in inches by 0.025. (Say, you are 5ft 5ins – that is 65ins × 0.025. You are 1.625 metres.)
- Square your height. (1.625 × 1.625 is 2.64.)
- Now divide your weight in kilograms by your squared height. (66.8 ÷ 2.64.)
- Your BMI is 25.3.

The international classification of BMIs is as follows:

Below 20: Underweight
20–25: Acceptable
25–30: Overweight
30–40: Obese
Above 40: Very obese

So, according to this, if your BMI is 25.3 you are only marginally overweight.

Work out *your* own BMI now and see how you do. If your figure is 30 or over, you can be pretty sure you could do with shedding some body fat even if your WHR wasn't much over average. While the heavy 'pear shape' may not carry as much risk of heart disease, you may get other health problems such as arthritis or varicose veins.

If your BMI is 30 or over and you *did* have a high WHR too, you should definitely begin shedding fat as soon as possible.

But if, like lots of people, your BMI is somewhere between 25 and 30, you can decide whether or not you really need to lose much fat by looking at your WHR. If it was average or below average you probably don't need to shed any fat. If it was above average, you probably do!

In other words – the more inches you can pinch round your middle, the more important it is for you to lose fat. If you are a marginally overweight pear, you needn't worry so much.

Try the WHR and BMI once a month or so, while you shed fat and step up your activity levels, and see how they alter. They are a good guide for telling you when your body is back in shape!

Right now – if you've decided you really need to attack that fat and get fit – turn the page and let's start. You'll find out how *Fat Attack* helps you to achieve just that.

CHAPTER 2

Fat Cutting Without Fuss

Just *why* do we eat so much fat?

According to the most recent nationwide survey of our eating habits, two-thirds of us know that it would be a good idea to cut down our fat intake, both for our health and for our waistlines. And yet, as a nation, we are eating just as much fat – and as much saturated fat – as ever.

One reason is that, perhaps surprisingly, most of us still aren't sure which the high-fat foods are – we especially want more information about the 'hidden' fats.

The other reason discovered by the survey – and confirmed by my own research – is that people are reluctant to swop to a lower-fat diet because the promise of a leaner body and better health isn't sufficient motivation to make up for what we see as the huge disadvantages that low-fat eating will bring.

In detail, these are the five problems we believe are associated with a low-fat diet:

- We are worried that a low-fat diet will leave us feeling hungry and dissatisfied.
- We are convinced that a low-fat diet will taste bland and boring.

- We believe that healthier, low-fat eating will be more expensive.
- We believe that a low-fat diet will take longer to plan, shop for, prepare and cook than our usual diet.
- We are reluctant in any event to change the eating habits of a lifetime.

On the face of it, these seem like valid reasons. But, fortunately, a healthy, reduced-fat diet doesn't have to involve all these disadvantages – or, indeed, any of them.

Believe me, you can eat a delicious diet, based on the kinds of food you already eat and enjoy, and still reduce your fat levels to well within official guidelines.

I don't believe in drastic solutions. There is no point in dictating to you what to do and what to eat if you can't stick to it! We all want to enjoy our food. Well, I am sure that by following the *Fat Attack* way of eating you will actually enjoy your food *more* – because eating is even *more* pleasurable if you can enjoy it without feeling guilty, as so many people do, knowing all the time that they are not doing themselves any favours with less-than-healthy choices.

One of the reasons I have been able to achieve a reduced-fat plan that you will enjoy is that I haven't gone over the top on fat reduction. In *Fat Attack* you'll find no fat-*free* recipes or *very* low-fat menus. If we reduce our saturated fat there is no need to make major alterations to our intake of other fats. There is no *need* to go any lower than 20–25 per cent fat in our diets (for fat loss) or 30 per cent (for weight maintenance). So you don't have to kiss all your favourite foods goodbye – and that's a promise.

In this chapter we're going to look more closely at the hidden fats that still seem to confuse many of us. And then, one by one, I am going to explain how we avoid your five major objections to a low-fat diet.

FAT IN DISGUISE

Many people who follow what they imagine is a typical slimming diet are horrified to find out that they've been eating loads of well-hidden fat!

How many times do I see people refuse the dessert trolley offerings and instead plump for an incredibly high-fat plateful of cheese and crackers?

How many times do I still see people choose the salad option at a café, not realizing that their saintly salad is stuffed with fat in the form of coleslaw, potato salad and mayonnaise or vinaigrette dressing – all high-fat foods that turn lettuce and cottage cheese into a dieter's nightmare!

I'm not saying you can't eat cheese, or coleslaw, etc. But it pays to know where the fat in your food is, so that you can incorporate the high-fat foods into your diet in a sensible way, or find ways to replace them.

Finding the fat

The *Fat Attack* 30-day plan is your ideal starting place because I've done all the hard work in finding and eliminating unnecessary fat from your diet. After 30 days on this plan you will almost instinctively know what is low-fat and what isn't. After the 30 days are up you can repeat them as many times as you like, but for even freer eating you'll want to devise your own diet. I go into this in more detail in chapter 7.

Most pre-packed food gives fat content on its packaging and this, too, can be helpful. However, I'd like to give you a quick word of warning about the fat content information on such foods. In this book when we talk about total fat intake per day of 20, 25 or 30 per cent, we are talking in terms of percentage of total *calories* in your diet. But, usually, the fat content of a commercial product is listed in grams per 100g; in other words, the percentage of the total *weight* of the product. Because much of the weight of any food product is water, which is calorie-free, this gives you a misleading low impression of fat content.

To work out the correct information all you do is multiply the number of fat grams per 100g by 9 (each gram contains 9 calories) and work out that figure as a percentage of the total calories per 100g. For instance, a ready-made salad contains the following per 100g: 10g fat and 205 calories. 10g fat = 90 calories. Then, using a calculator, punch in 90 ÷ 205 per cent. The answer is 43.9 – meaning that just under 44 per cent of the total calories of the product are fat calories. The manufacturer will call this product '10 per cent fat' (because the fat content *is* 10 per cent of the total weight) – I'd call it (and you should call it) a high-fat food at 44 per cent.

Let's have a quick rundown of the major sources of saturated fat in your diet – the foods that I am going to show you how to eat less of without pain.

Remember, we're cutting the fat, not the food!

- High-fat (at least 35 per cent of total calories) *protein* foods include: bacon, most kinds of beef, chicken with skin, duck, ham, lamb, liver, meat loaf, pork, sausages, pâté, some kinds of fish fried in batter, whole milk, all cheese except diet cottage cheese, eggs, whole-milk yogurts and full-fat fromage frais.

- High-fat *carbohydrate* foods include: some chips (depending on how they are cooked), doughnuts, sponge and other cake, croissants, biscuits, some cereal bars, pasties, most kinds of pastry, some savoury snacks and canned cream of tomato soup.
- High-fat items that you add to food yourself in cooking or at table include: butter, many margarines, lard, suet, salad cream and mayonnaise, cream, and sauces made from whole milk.
- High-fat sweet and dessert items include: chocolate, toffees, standard ice cream, cheesecakes, gâteaux, fruit pies, pastries, canned puddings.
- High-fat ready meals include: many, such as lasagnes, curries, moussakas, satays, mornays.

If you are thinking, 'Well, that list includes all my favourites so what is she talking about?' please do believe me when I say you *can* eat all those types of foods, but in the next few pages I will show you how we are going to attack the *fat* in them, or alter the *proportions* in the rest of your diet to make it lower in fat overall.

By the way, there are other high-fat items that haven't been included on the above lists because they are not high in *saturated* fat. Foods such as olive and corn oil, fishes, some spreads, nuts and avocados, for instance.

Now let's tackle those objections!

OBJECTION: A LOW-FAT DIET WILL LEAVE ME HUNGRY AND DISSATISFIED

In chapter 1, I explained how trials on both sides of the Atlantic had shown that people who follow a diet containing 20–25 per cent fat seem to be able to shed weight steadily while eating their fill of the 'complex' carbohydrate foods. Because it is largely these carbohydrate foods that make you feel full – and stave off hunger pangs between meals – you *won't* feel hungry on *Fat Attack*.

There is no question of anyone on the *Fat Attack* plan having small portions of 'diet' food on their plates. What you will be eating are meals with controlled amounts of fat, but plenty of the complex carbohydrates, which are, simply, bread, potatoes, rice and other grains, pasta, cereals, pulses, fruit and vegetables.

There will be no need to weigh any of these foods. All you need do is follow my guidelines in chapter 4 on what are 'sensible', 'average' or 'large' portion sizes.

You *don't* have less food on your plate than someone who isn't on a fat loss plan. All we are doing is altering the balance – more carbohydrates, less fat. So, because, as we have seen, weight for weight, fat is so much more calorific than carbohydrate, you will be reducing not only the fat, but also the calories, in your diet quite dramatically.

That is why the *Fat Attack* system is the perfect fat- and weight-loss plan for people who have failed on typical 'lettuce and cottage cheese' diets in the past.

Here are some examples of high-fat meals followed by their lower-fat counterparts. The reduced-fat meals weigh the same (or more) as the high-fat meals, but have far fewer calories and a fraction of the fat!

Note: Remember, there are 9 calories in every gram of fat.

Roast lamb – high fat

	calories	*grams of fat*
• 110g (4oz) roast shoulder of lamb	320	26.0
• 2 medium chunks (150g, 5½ oz) potato roasted in the lamb fat	235	7.2
• 150g (5½ oz) onion sauce, traditional	150	6.4
• small portion (50g, 2oz) peas	27	0.35
• small portion (50g, 2oz) carrots	11	0.0
• 3 tablespoons (60g, 2oz) pan gravy	45	4.0
• 2 teaspoons mint sauce	10	0.0

Total weight of meal: 580g (1¼ lb)
Total calories: 798
Total fat: 44g
(There are then 396 fat calories in this meal, which is 50 per cent of total calories.)

Roast lamb – low fat

	calories	*grams of fat*
• 80g (3oz) lean roast leg of lamb	144	6.0
• 3 average (200g, 7oz) new potatoes, brushed with olive oil and dry roasted	200	5.0
• 150g (5½ oz) onion sauce made following recipe on page 100	76	2.5
• medium portion (75g, 3oz) peas	51	0.7
• medium to large portion (100g, 3½ oz) carrots	23	trace
• 3 tablespoons (60g, 2oz) well-skimmed pan gravy	20	1.5
• 2 teaspoons mint sauce	10	0.0

Total weight of meal: 680g ($1^1/_2$ lb)
Total calories: 524
Total fat: 15.7g
(There are then 141 fat calories in this meal, which is 27 per cent of total calories.)

Baked chicken – high fat

	calories	*grams of fat*
• Average portion (200g, 7oz) chicken breast, baked with skin	225	15.0
• 225g (8oz) baked potato	190	0.2
• 15g ($^1/_2$ oz) butter to top potato	111	12.3
• small portion (100g, $3^1/_2$ oz) courgettes, sautéed in 1 tablespoon oil	140	15.4
• small portion (50g, $1^3/_4$ oz) sweetcorn	63	2.0
• 3 tablespoons (60g, 2oz) instant gravy	21	0.0

Total weight of meal: 665g ($1^1/_2$ lb)
Total calories: 750
Total fat: 45g
(There are then 405 fat calories in this meal, which is 54 per cent of the total calories.)

Baked chicken – low fat

	calories	*grams of fat*
• 1 average (125g, $4^1/_2$ oz) skinned breast of chicken fillet, coated in barbecue seasoning and baked	150	5.0
• large (275g, 10oz) baked potato	232	0.3
• 1 level tablespoon Kraft fat free mayonnaise to top potato	10	0.0

• medium portion (125g, 4½ oz) courgettes,	25	0.5
simmered in Passata with herbs	20	0.0
• small portion (50g, 2oz) sweetcorn	63	2.0
• 2 tablespoons (40g, 1½ oz) instant gravy (Bovril granules)	15	0.0

Total weight of meal: 670g (1½ lb)
Total calories: 515
Total fat: 8g
(There are then 72 fat calories in this meal, which is 14 per cent of the total calories.)

So *now* you can see how you can shed body fat without hunger – by shedding that fat from your food! It's easy the *Fat Attack* way!

OBJECTION: A LOW-FAT DIET WILL TASTE BLAND AND BORING

If you have tried low-fat eating before and have given up because it was too monotonous and tasteless for you, I do understand. Some low-fat diets are just that. But they needn't be. The daily menus and recipes in this book prove that. And people who try the menus say time and again how surprised they are that the food is so good to eat.

I have achieved this in several ways – easy ways that you can copy just as easily and with just as good results.

• I hardly ever just take away fat without adding something *better* in its place! You saw examples in the comparative meals just now. The low-fat baked chicken dinner is, to my mind, far tastier than the high-fat one because the chicken is cooked with barbecue seasoning rather than plain; the potato has a delicious creamy mayonnaise-style topping rather than just a lump of fat; and the courgettes are cooked in a delicious sauce rather than just fried in oil.

• I've made full use of tasty ingredients such as mushrooms, onions, garlic, soya sauce, spices, Worcestershire sauce, all kinds of seasonings – you name it, I've tried it on your behalf. And anything that didn't pass my own taste test – I didn't include!

• Cashing in unashamedly on our current, and growing, love of tastes from all corners of the world, I've included plenty of ethnic foods for you to try if you like – Mexican, Chinese, Thai, Indian, American, Mediterranean – all those influences are there and, luckily for us, it's very easy to cook many delicious ethnic dishes keeping the fat content low and the taste factor high! You don't *have* to eat all these foods on the 30-day plan – but you can't complain there are no interesting meals!

• I have not replaced a high-fat ingredient or item with a lower-fat one unless the lower-fat one performs equally well in taste terms. There are many, many reduced- or low-fat foods that do taste just as good as their high-fat counterparts. For example, low-fat crème fraîche is just as creamy and lovely as ordinary crème fraîche, low-fat Bio yogurt is just as delicious as whole-milk Bio yogurt. These are the kinds of swaps I promise you you won't notice, and yet they can save masses of fat and calories every day.

• I've experimented with various cooking methods and used most often the ones that enhance the flavour of the food – for instance, dry-roasted vegetables taste marvellous. Cooking in foil parcels keeps all those wonderful flavours and aromas; and clever low-fat frying is another of my favourite methods. People add, usually without thinking about it, ounces of fat almost daily in their cooking, most of which isn't necessary for flavour. I always include enough fat to make a dish taste great if it needs it – but no more. And in swopping saturated fat for unsaturated fats in cooking I'm making the dishes healthier too.

OBJECTION: A LOW-FAT DIET WILL BE EXPENSIVE

Far from costing you more, a reduced-fat diet can actually cut your food bills.

I think it is quite appalling how many of us really believe that 'diet' foods and 'health' foods are so expensive. OK, some low-calorie foods can be pricey – lobster and out-of-season strawberries may be the costliest diet on earth! But you don't have to eat them. And certainly not on the *Fat Attack* plan.

Fat Attack helps you save money in three ways:

- As you've seen, you won't be eating less but you will be altering the balance of foods on your plate. The foods you are going to be eating *more* of tend to be the lowest-cost ones – that is, bread, potatoes, rice, pasta, cereals, and pulses. At first glance, you may think some of the low-fat meals include more expensive items, but usually it doesn't work out this way at all. For example, in the low-fat roast lamb meal I have used as an example on page 23, yes – leg of lamb is dearer than shoulder. But you will see I've altered the balance on your plate so that you have a smaller quantity of lamb, which will work out no more expensive than the portion of shoulder in the high-fat meal. Also, it is usually true that the cheaper, fatty cuts tend to 'shrink' more than leaner meat when you cook them, so that a lot of your bargain joint ends up down the sink.

- There is plenty of choice every day on the plan so that you can buy whichever alternative is least expensive, if you want to. This allows you to take advantage of bargains as and when you see them. I have included a few more expensive items, such as steak and prawns, in the plan, but there is no obligation to buy them. As an alternative to steak, for instance, you could have burger; as an alternative to prawns you could have hard-boiled egg!
- Many people cite fresh fruit and vegetables as being expensive and it is certainly true that I want you to eat plenty of these – probably more than you have been eating up to now. But I deliberately don't dictate exactly which you should eat so that again you can make full use of the ones in season, special offers, bulk buys etc. Again, you can choose exotic fruits and expensive vegetables if you want – but there is no need. And if you buy in bulk or in season you can freeze the surplus; or, if you have any spare garden space, why not try to grow some of your own? It's a great hobby and beats couch potato-ing!

OBJECTION: A LOW-FAT DIET WILL TAKE UP TOO MUCH TIME

The *Fat Attack* eating plan is designed for ordinary people leading typical, busy lives. As far as possible, I have eliminated all the fuss and bother that goes with many diet plans. This is how I've done it:

- I've kept recipes optional and, in the main, simple and quick to cook. There are easy alternatives to every recipe at each meal.
- I have kept weighing and measuring to an absolute minimum. As explained earlier, there is no strict portion control of the complex carbohydrate foods, so no more weighing a slice of bread or a baked potato or a bowl of breakfast cereal! Where possible, I've used everyday measures such as tablespoons, as well as giving weights.
- I've ensured that the plan is suitable for almost everyone, so that there will be no need to prepare different meals for other members of the family. Men, as well as women, will enjoy the plan – and people who don't need to lose any body fat can add on calories in the form of extra complex carbohydrates (more detail on that in chapter 4).
- There are plenty of convenience foods included in the diet – for example, baked beans, instant mash, frozen vegetables. In fact, many of the healthiest low-fat foods are also the most convenient! What could be easier to prepare than a sandwich or a baked potato? What is quicker to grab than a banana or an apple? What speedier breakfast than a bowl of cereal, or faster dessert than a yogurt or low-fat ice cream?
- If your time is precious and you are not so worried about cost, these days almost any healthy food can be bought ready prepared – for instance, mixed salads, stir-fry mixtures or even oranges peeled, segmented and ready to eat! Busy people may find these short cuts well worth the extra expense.

Lastly, if you have always been the type of person who wants anything to eat as long as it's quick and easy – can

I leave you with a thought? Eating food should be a pleasure. There is a lot of enjoyment to be found in choosing and preparing your own meals; in producing something yourself. So if you resent any time at all spent on food, perhaps it is time to have a rethink of your priorities. Why not relax a bit, start to make more time for the kitchen and for giving yourself (and your family if you have one) attractive platefuls of real food? Who knows? – it could change your life.

OBJECTION: I DON'T WANT TO CHANGE THE EATING HABITS OF A LIFETIME!

If you have eaten in a certain way for years, of course the thought of suddenly having to throw all that out and start learning totally new eating habits is bound to be something you view with suspicion and dread – and will probably reject.

That is why *Fat Attack* does *not* ask you to make *drastic* changes. I am not extreme in my views or my advice. I don't ask you to sit down to a plate of raw beansprouts and tofu for your lunch; or to tuck in to a nut cutlet with brown rice for your supper if you've been a red meat and mashed potatoes person all your life. I am not going to suggest you give up your cups of tea and coffee for herbal brews; or make you chuck out the white bread and eat only stoneground wholemeal. To shed body fat and to give your heart a healthier chance you don't *need* to do any of that. No one food or drink is either forbidden or obligatory.

All we are going to do is (yes, I'll say it again!) *alter the balance* of what is on your plate – less (sometimes just a little less) of the high-fat foods and more of the high-carbohydrate foods. (Your protein intake will stay roughly the same as it was before without you having to worry about that.)

We will *make swops*, using low- or lower-fat versions of high-fat foods, that you won't even notice.

And we will *cook clever*, turning traditional high-fat delights such as curries and Bolognese sauce into low-fat treats with no loss of taste. I repeat, there is *no need* to give up all the things you like best. You just need to cook them in a slightly different way which will become second nature within a week or two.

Lastly, the menus in *Fat Attack* take account of your own likes and dislikes so you are never stuck with 'having to' eat any one particular meal or food you detest.

In the next chapter we take a closer look at some of the food cravings that you may think will hinder your plans to shed body fat – things like chocolate, and chips!

CHAPTER 3

Fat Addictions – and How to Handle Them

Everyone's different – but there are certain foods, and types of foods, that crop up time and again when I talk to people trying to cut down their fat intake and lose weight.

'It'd be all right but for the chocolate,' say many. 'I just love it and I don't see how I'm going to give it up.'

'Ah – I'm a cheesaholic,' said one man. 'Life without cheese would hardly be worth living!'

But, as you'll soon see, you don't actually have to learn to live totally without those favourite foods. So here, one by one, we'll look at the most typical high-fat binge foods and see how we can 'alter the balance' again, without causing you misery.

CHOCOLATE

Almost everyone enjoys chocolate. Some people can open a pack of chocolate and eat only a little bit, while to others this would seem impossible.

Some people eat so much of the stuff that they not only feel controlled by it, but also have a weight problem.

I'm not going to ask you to give up chocolate. All I would like to do, if you are the type who eats tons of it, is to turn you into someone who can enjoy your chocolate in reasonable quantities within your healthier reduced-fat diet. According to my research, there are four main reasons why people eat too much chocolate.

1 Low blood sugar

People who say they crave chocolate frequently are often those who either have erratic eating patterns (particularly, skipping meals) or eat a fairly poor diet, nutritionally. Such people often find themselves bingeing on sweet food – and often that sweet food is chocolate.

The craving for something sweet may come about because of low blood sugar levels (hypoglycaemia). This can occur when a meal, snack or drink containing a high level of 'simple' carbohydrate (i.e. sugar or glucose) has been taken – say, a large quantity of chocolate, or a sugary drink such as cola or alcohol.

Such a meal, snack or drink, especially taken on an 'empty stomach' may stimulate the pancreas to produce large quantities of insulin in order to cope with the sudden rise in blood sugar. This can leave an insulin residue which then pushes the blood sugar levels down *low*, and at this stage you may have that sweet food craving.

Because chocolate, with its high simple-sugar content, is so easily available and widely advertised it is often the food that comes to mind.

But if you succumb and have that chocolate (or, indeed, another meal, snack or drink high in the 'simple' carbohydrates) you'll start the whole process off again!

Foods high in the 'complex' carbohydrates such as wholemeal bread, potatoes, baked beans, and so on, don't have this effect.

2 Habit

If you've been a regular chocolate eater since early childhood, it's an ingrained habit. And any habit can be hard to break, especially if it's a pleasant one – albeit with its downside! Habitual chocolate eaters will 'always' have a chocolate wafer with their morning coffee and a couple of chocolate digestives with a late-night drink. They don't particularly consider whether they're really enjoying this habit – they just do it.

3 Comfort

People who find themselves depressed, miserable, bored, lonely, let down or irritated in one way or another often seek refuge in chocolate. If we like chocolate it can seem like a real cheer-me-up if we're down. This may not be purely psychological – chocolate contains the stimulant caffeine (in small quantities) as well as phenylethylamine – a chemical similar to one produced in the brain when we are in love!

4 Reward

How many times as a child were you given chocolate or sweets to reward good behaviour? It's a pattern that remains with many of us into adulthood. We award ourselves a big bar of chocolate after a particularly tough day in the office. We go for a long walk and our reward for being so energetic is a chocolate bar. And so on.

Some of these reasons are interlinked – for instance, that chocolate bought after a long walk is perhaps part reward, part because your blood sugar level is low through exercising hard and not having eaten for a long time. But virtually all chocolate eating can be classed in one or more of the above categories.

Now, I would like you, if you are a chocolate lover, to keep a 'chocolate log' for the next few days – a week or more if you can. Your chocolate diary should record the date and time you eat chocolate (including things like chocolate mousse or cake) and the reason why you ate it. Try to be honest and to think carefully about those reasons. The first thing you think of is often not the truth of the matter. Write down your reason, and anything else about that chocolate-eating session that occurs to you. How you felt during and after it, for example. Then note down which of the above four categories it came into. There may be more than one.

When you've completed several days of your diary you will begin to see what it is that drives you to eat chocolate most frequently. Whether it's one main reason, or a mix of all four, it will help. Once you know what triggers a chocolate-eating session, you can do something about it.

Here are the solutions.

Controlling low blood sugar

You'll be pleased to hear that the *Fat Attack* diet plan will almost certainly cure this problem. This is because it asks you to eat regularly, and contains plenty of the complex carbohydrates that fill you up and keep your blood sugar level constant as they take a long time to be completely absorbed, so that the release of insulin and the conversion of carbohydrate to glucose is slow and steady, which is the way it should be. This will stop the 'highs and lows' that come with poor eating habits and a diet high in refined sugar.

The first rule is: never let yourself get so hungry that you end up on a chocolate binge, don't skip meals, and eat everything you are allowed at each meal.

And rule two is: never satisfy your hunger with chocolate, or any other simple carbohydrate food such as sweets or sugary biscuits. Eat a snack (or meal if it's mealtime) that contains some complex carbohydrate (e.g. a piece of bread, a rye crispbread, a cold potato, an apple, or a couple of spoonfuls of baked beans).

Getting into the right habits

Your chocolate diary can help you here, too, by showing you the times you habitually eat chocolate. The solution then is to decide beforehand what you are going to eat or do instead of eating that chocolate bar. This is best done in two stages.

Stage one is to substitute what you normally eat with something still sweet or chocolatey, but lower in fat and calories, or with half the usual amount plus a healthier choice. For example, you usually have a four-finger KitKat with your morning coffee. Make it a two-finger KitKat plus an apple. Or you usually have two chocolate digestives at teatime. Have a Lo Bar. A Mars bar will set you back 300 calories and 9 grams of fat, but two slices of malt loaf with low-fat spread would be just as satisfying but only 150 calories and 3 or 4 grams of fat. To get out of the 'habit' mentally, choose something different as often as possible (see Chocolate Box on page 38).

Stage two is to begin to think of new habits to fill up the time you would have been eating. With your cup of tea, why not buy a paper instead of a chocolate bar and enjoy that? Do the crossword or quiz. Or have a cold drink instead of tea or coffee and go for a 15-minute walk.

I'm not saying you can't have chocolate, remember – within the *Fat Attack* 30-day plan you can choose chocolate every day if you want to for your treat. But if you are just eating lots of it out of habit you may find it easier than you thought possible to cut down – and save yourself masses of calories and fat!

Beat the urge to comfort eat

Much comfort eating is done at home, so the first stage is exactly the same as for habit eating: make swops in what you buy, so that there is less potential for damage.

Go shopping when your resolve is good (after a meal, usually) and be careful not to kid yourself about what you are putting in your shopping basket. Are those chocolate bars and biscuits really for the children? Don't you usually eat most of them instead? Will your partner really not be able to live without that double chocolate gâteau?

Step two is to find comforters other than chocolate for your 'down' times. Here are some suggestions:

• telephone a friend or relative • write a letter to someone who understands you • put on some music and dance • go out for a walk (exercise can lift stress and put you in a better mood) • look through your old photo albums or read your old diary • have a soak in the bath with a magazine or favourite book • wash your hair.

Comfort eating isn't easy to beat quickly but, again, your chocolate diary should help forewarn you about times when you are likely to do it, so if you pre-plan a strategy you can get it under control. The trouble with eating for comfort is that it is only a very fleeting comforter – next day you may feel guilty and in the long term even more fed up if it is making you pile on the stones.

Rewards you can really appreciate

There is no need to give up the idea of rewarding yourself (or letting the people who care about you reward you, come to that).

But if chocolate has been your typical reward, see what different 'prizes' you can give yourself as well. Think of a list of things you like that you might regard as small luxuries. Here's mine:

• A bunch of flowers • Some bulbs or plants for the window box – or a packet of seeds • A nice pair of silky tights or stockings • A glossy magazine • A bestselling paperback • A punnet of strawberries

Chocolate box

Swop any of these…	*For any of these…*
Bars	
KitKat (245)	Halo (95)
Mars (295)	Flake (170)
Boost (295	Lo Bar (100)
Snickers (300)	Milky Way (120)
Caramel (245)	Boots Shapers Caramel (100)
Ice cream and desserts	
Choc 'n nut Cornetto (210)	Choc ice bar (120)
Chocolate cheesecake (300)	2 chocolate ice cream scoops (150)

Chocolate pot (300)
Profiteroles (400)
Frozen choc mousse (100)
Chocolate Puddi (115)

Biscuits and cakes
Chocolate digestive (85)
Choc chip cookie (40)
Chocolate gâteau or fudge cake (400)
Dairy Cream Eclair (120)
Chocolate donut (300)
Chocolate cup cake (130)

Chocolate drink
Standard hot chocolate (200)
Ovaltine Options (40)

Figures in brackets = number of calories

CHEESE

If you're hooked on cheese, it's a long way from being all bad news. Cheese is a wonderful source of calcium, protein and vitamins, as well as being so versatile in cooking that it would be a terrible shame to try to ban cheese from your shopping list. And don't worry, I'm not going to!

The thing you've got to be aware of, though, is that most cheeses are dense, rich dairy foods, high in saturated fats. The trick, then, is to cut your cheese intake down to reasonable levels while still getting all cheese's goodness and that tangy, savoury taste you crave.

I've done just that in the *Fat Attack* plan by the following methods, all of which you can use in the future.

- Whenever possible, select a lower-fat, lower-calorie cheese in place of a higher-fat, higher-calorie one. The highest-fat, highest-calorie cheeses are traditional Cheddar, Stilton, blue Brie (Cambozola), full-fat cream cheese, blue Cheshire, and blue Wensleydale. All these contain at least 75 per cent fat and at least 120 calories per ounce. Some tasty, lower-fat, lower-calorie alternatives are Brie, Camembert, Bresse Bleu, feta, Danish blue, Edam, mozzarella, and Port Salut. These all contain 70–95 calories an ounce and less fat.

- Use 'reduced-fat' versions of your favourite cheeses whenever possible. You can get reduced-fat Cheddar and many other types – the Cheddar, for instance, contains only around 70 calories per ounce as opposed to 120 for the full-fat version. Not everyone enjoys these reduced-fat cheeses, but some taste much better than others and have a better texture than others, so try a few until you find one you do like – and bear in mind that even if you only use them in cooking (say in a cheese sauce) you will be saving lots of saturated fat over the months.
- If it's the tang of cheese you want, you may find that you will be satisfied with a small piece of the strongest mature Cheddar or Stilton – say an ounce, which represents 120–130 calories – whereas if you buy the mild Cheddar you may need 2–3 ounces (up to 360 calories) for the same effect.
- When offered a cheeseboard in a restaurant or at someone's house, ask the host or waiter to cut you just a small bit of your favourite. If the board is left with you, you will choose several and keep coming back for more!
- For salads and sandwiches, always grate your cheese. It looks much more – and it takes longer to eat. In a salad, you can mix your grated cheese half and half with grated carrot for an even bigger plateful which tastes great.
- When you need cheese to be sliced, use a special cheese slicer, available from hardware shops, which will slice it really thin, and again it looks more.

• If you enjoy cheese spread, do try some of the low-fat versions. St Ivel Shape is particularly good, and if you're using it on crispbreads or in sandwiches you can forget the low-fat spread because you won't need any, thus saving more fat and calories.

• Make full use of pre-portioned cheeses. Camembert often comes in its own little triangles which make a perfect portion for a lunch; or the pick-and-mix selections at the supermarket will give you plenty of choice.

• If it is the cheesy taste you are after, you can get it in several ways without actually eating cheese. Here are some ideas:

1 cheese thin savoury biscuit (15 calories)
1oz (25g) slice cheese bread (90 calories)
1 pack Cheesy Wotsits (110 calories)
1 pack KP Cheese Crunches (75 calories)
1 pack Cheese Quavers (95 calories)

• In cooking, cheese goes a long way, so get the taste by cooking pizzas, bakes topped with low-calorie cheese sauce (recipes for both in chapter 5) and dishes sprinkled with Parmesan (only 30 calories per tablespoon).

FRYING WITH LESS FAT

If you're cutting fat, will the frying pan have to go? The short answer is that is no – it won't. If most of your meals to date have been straight out of a frying pan, and you think of fried food in terms of a sausage wallowing in half an inch of lard or crinkle-cut chips fried twice before serving, then yes, there is a little rethinking to be done. But food cooked in the frying pan is perfectly acceptable as part of your reduced-fat diet. Before frying, always think, 'Is there a better method of cooking this food?'

Remember you can get the fried taste with a fraction of the fat and calories. Here are your guidelines for frying.

Utensils

For cooking the *Fat Attack* way, your frying pan needs to be the best-quality, heaviest pan you can afford and it needs to be non-stick. With a good, non-stick pan you can reduce cooking fat down to a minimum.

There are four other types of pan that are useful for healthier fry-type cooking.

The first is a *griddle pan* – a large, square or round sheet with a very shallow lip round the edge and often with ridges across it every inch or so, so that you can griddle steak, sausages, etc., and the fat drips out and runs to the bottom, leaving the food high and dry on the ridges. Food cooked this way is delicious. It's a bit like barbecuing, and also ideal for firm cuts of fish.

Next is a *covered 'dry-fry' pan*. This is a pan with a lid and a central funnel. You add a very small amount of oil plus your food and the food cooks in a combination of fat and dry heat or, if what you are cooking has a reasonable water content, steam heat.

Then there is, of course, the *wok* – the steep-sided large pan essential in Chinese cooking and incredibly useful for all types of British cooking, too! The special shape ensures you can keep stirring without the food falling out; the heat is evenly distributed so the contents cook quickly. You can get electric woks as well as ones you simply rest over the hob.

Lastly, I wouldn't be without a smallish, non-stick *omelette pan* with rounded sides, kept especially for omelette-making. This, then, just needs the merest brushing of oil or butter before heating and using. After use, it should only be wiped clean with kitchen paper, never immersed in water, or next time your omelette will stick!

The last utensil you will need is a cook's heatproof brush.

Fats for frying

I'll be honest with you – I would prefer that you ditch lard altogether as it really is adding unnecessary saturated fat to your diet. Vegetable oils achieve a good taste for almost any dish, with the possible exception of omelettes when a little butter always seems to be called for.

I would also prefer you not to use hard margarines, which are high in the trans fatty acids and certainly add no more flavour than the best vegetable oils.

So try to get into the habit of using pure vegetable oils for frying. I like to have a small collection because different oils often suit different purposes.

I like *olive oil* for stir-frying onions (a method frequently used in the recipe section) in soups, casseroles, bakes, etc. The lighter, paler olive oils are best for this. Corn, sunflower, rapeseed or safflower make perfectly good substitutes, though as olive oil and rapeseed oil are higher in mono-unsaturates and the others are higher in poly-unsaturates, it is good to use both types in your cooking. Groundnut (peanut) oil is great for Thai and Indonesian dishes, while sesame oil is superb in Chinese dishes. It is also worth buying a spray can of Fry Light for 'dry-frying'.

Methods

Here are my four tried-and-tested methods for frying, one of which will suit any food, any recipe and any occasion.

Completely dry-frying Using your good-quality non-stick pan or griddle, simply add your food to the pan, turn on the heat and gradually increase it as the foods begins to cook in its own fat. Don't turn or move the meat until it's had a chance to brown, otherwise it may stick.

This method is ideal for minced meat, sausages and bacon – all foods that, even if you choose the 'extra-lean' variety, contain enough fat to fry themselves. If you then pour away any fat which melts off the meat, you will be cutting even more fat from your diet.

Brush-on frying Again, using a decent non-stick pan or griddle, simply coat the pan with the thinnest of oil or butter coatings, using a brush dipped into the oil or melted butter in a saucer. You could also use your Fry Light spray, if you have one, for a similar result.

This method works well with steaks, pancakes, omelettes, 'fried' eggs and oily fish such as salmon. The food only needs turning once, halfway through, including the 'fried' eggs. Unlike completely dry-frying, you should heat your pan up first then add the food so it browns immediately.

Stir-frying Put a little oil in the pan (a teaspoonful to a tablespoonful depending on the amount of food you're cooking), heat it and add your finely sliced food, putting the things that take longest to cook in first, and stirring constantly. Later you may add stock or a sauce or even a little water to prevent sticking. This method can be used not only for Chinese dishes but for side vegetables as a welcome change from boiling, and for all kinds of quick-cook dishes such as stroganoffs and Balti curries. It's ideal for all vegetables (as long as the tougher ones, such as carrots, are very thinly sliced), all poultry, all tender cuts of beef, all lamb and pork, and for the firmer fishes such as monkfish and shellfish.

There are many stir-fry recipes in chapter 5.

Shallow-frying This method uses a maximum of 1 tablespoon oil in a non-stick pan, and these days I mostly use it just for pre-cooking onions for a recipe dish or for sautéeing potatoes for a special treat. If you're cooking highly absorbent vegetables, such as mushrooms and aubergines, in oil, it is better to stir-fry them as that way they cook more quickly and the oil doesn't disappear in two seconds!

If shallow-fried vegetables do look as if they are drying out you can always add a little stock.

After shallow-frying, if there *is* any surplus fat it should be poured off and all suitable food should be patted or drained on kitchen paper to absorb excess oil.

If you use all or any of these methods as your regular way to fry food, then you won't feel guilty once in a blue moon for having a plate of deep-fried chips or fish – but once you've learnt to fry with less oil, you'll probably find the traditional way is just too, well – greasy!

Chip talk

As chips are the UK's most frequently consumed high-fat fried food, it's worth looking at how 'chip satisfaction' without all the fat and calories.

Obviously one answer is to use oven chips – the very lowest-fat kind you can get, which will certainly save you some fat, but not as much as you might think, as the chips are already part-cooked in fat when you buy them. Check the packet to make sure they are cooked in vegetable oil – preferably a pure oil.

If you are going to have real chips sometimes as your treat, you can still save masses of fat and calories by following these tips:

- Cut the chips as big as you can – they absorb less fat than smaller ones.
- Dry them well on kitchen paper before cooking.
- Use fresh corn oil and heat it to the correct temperature before adding the chips – if the oil isn't hot enough the chips will sit around and absorb more fat while they are waiting to begin cooking.
- Don't try cooking too many chips at one go as, again, this reduces the temperature of the oil and the chips will absorb extra fat.
- When cooked, drain and pat the chips on kitchen paper.
- Never twice-fry them.
- Make sure your cooking oil is fresh – if it looks a dark colour or has a film on it, the 'good for you' poly-unsaturates in it are busy turning themselves into not-so-good for you oxidized fats.

Roast chips You can make your own delicious oven chips this way. Choose medium-sized potatoes and leave the skins on. Scrub them clean and cut them lengthways into eights. Dry them very well. Brush with olive or corn oil and put on a baking tray. Sprinkle with salt and pepper and roast for 30 minutes, turning once – or until crisp, golden and tender. Yummy!

IS IT GOODBYE TO BAKES, PUDS AND PIES?

If your particular love is all kinds of pastry, or puddings and cake shop goodies, here are some tips and tricks.

Pies and puddings

- If you make your own pies, forget double crusts – instead choose a single layer, and make either flans or top-crust pies which will immediately save you masses of fat and calories.
- Use a deeper dish for your top-crust pies so that you have more filling – e.g. fruit – and less pastry per portion.
- Make sure the fillings are as low in fat as possible to compensate for the high-fat crust.
- Try using filo pastry instead of shortcrust or puff. Simply brush a very little oil on to each layer. The oil is better for you than the saturated fat that goes into most traditional pastry. Filo gives a delicious, crunchy result and is also ideal for tarts and flans.
- Try some alternative toppings sometimes. For savoury pies, use potato with a little grated cheese on top, or breadcrumbs mixed with Parmesan.
- For sweet pies, you can top with crushed breakfast cereal or traditional crumble mixture mixed half and half with porridge oats or muesli.
- Try making more puddings using bread rather than pastry – e.g. summer pudding or apple charlotte.

- For desserts, you can find plenty to choose from that isn't too high in fat – fromage frais, sorbets, jelly, low-calorie ice cream, all served with fresh or even canned fruit, for instance.

Bakes and cakes

Some people find the goodies in the cake shop and baker's more addictive than chocolate – and if you are a cake-o-holic rather than a chocoholic you can use many of the same strategies we covered in the chocolate section (see page 32). You don't have to give up your favourites, but remember that most bakery items hide a lot more fat than you'd think. Here are some useful swops you could make most of the time – all of them will satisfy you for far less fat and calories than their counterparts, so you can have a now-and-then treat of the more wicked items in the cake shop without having to worry.

Instead of these ...	*Try one of these ...*
Cream cake (250–300)	Large slice malt loaf (110)
Danish pastry (350)	Teacake with low-fat spread (170)
Croissant (280)	Crumpet with butter (125)
Jam doughnut (260)	Scotch pancake with syrup (120)
Fruit scone with jam and cream (250)	Large slice fruit bread with low-sugar jam and aerosol cream (120)
Fresh fruit tart with confectioner's custard (300)	Fresh fruit tart with pure fruit spread (140)

CHAPTER 4

The 30-Day **fat***attack* Diet

The 30-day plan puts into practice all the advice and tips that you've learnt in the past chapters. You will find it pleasant and easy to follow, especially as I've kept weighing and measuring to a minimum. There is plenty of choice at every meal and the plan is suitable for the whole family. If you don't need to shed fat, read the advice on page 51. I have included some notes on feeding children on this page too.

WHAT THE **fat***attack* DIET PLAN WILL DO FOR YOU

If you follow the plan as laid out, you will shed body fat. It will give you an average weight loss over the 30 days of between 8 and 12 lbs (3.6 and 5.4 kg) for women, and between 10 lbs and a stone (4.6 and 6.4 kg) for men. In general, the more surplus body fat you are currently carrying, the more pounds you will see disappearing during the 30 days.

If at the end of 30 days you still have more body fat to lose, you can safely repeat the programme until you are happy with your size.

You will see best fat loss if you combine the diet plan with regular exercise (see chapter 6, or the *Fat Attack* video).

Because the plan cuts saturated fat and includes enough of the 'good for you' fats, it is healthy and, if followed over a period of time, can offer real protection against heart disease.

Note: If you dislike fish, particularly oily fish, and don't intend to include it in your diet at least two or three times a week, you may consider supplementing the diet with a daily Omega-3 fish oil capsule (available from chemists).

The health benefits of the *Fat Attack* diet plan are enhanced by including all the other known nutritional heart protection factors:

- ***It is high in the 'ACE' vitamins*** – beta-carotene (a form of vitamin A found only in fruits and vegetables, particularly dark green, orange and yellow ones); vitamin C, found mainly in fruits and vegetables, and vitamin E, found mainly in vegetable oils, nuts, seeds, whole grains, leafy green vegetables and avocados.
- ***The fibre content*** of the diet is high, and five portions of fruit or vegetables a day are included, as recommended by the DoH and the WHO.
- ***There is plenty of soluble fibre*** – the kind, found mainly in oats and pulses, that can lower blood cholesterol.
- ***Garlic and moderate amounts of wine*** are two optional extras on the diet plan – both are known to have beneficial effects on the circulation and heart.
- ***The salt content*** of the plan is moderate to low, and a high salt intake is a known risk factor in high blood pressure.

Special instructions for men

If you have just a little fat to lose and/or are shorter than average, you can follow the basic plan. If you have much weight to lose or are much taller than average, you should substitute large portions of any carbohydrate food every time an 'average' portion is mentioned. That is, bread, potatoes, rice and grains, pasta, breakfast cereals and pulses. You can also add one extra *treat* a day plus an extra 150ml ($^1/_4$ pint) skimmed or semi-skimmed milk.

Special instructions for weight maintenance

If you don't need to lose any body fat but would like to follow the plan, simply increase portion sizes of all foods mentioned by around 25 per cent. If you need to eat still more to maintain your weight (say, because you are male), then increase the carbohydrate food portions still further – that is, bread, potatoes, rice and grains, pasta, breakfast cereals and pulses.

If you would like to maintain your weight and devise your own menus following the *Fat Attack* principles, then turn to chapter 7. However, I would suggest not doing this until you have followed the 30-day plan for at least one complete cycle, as it gets you into the habit of eating right.

Special instructions for feeding children

- Children under 5 should be given whole milk, not skimmed.
- Children of all ages should have at least 275ml ($^1/_2$pint) milk allowance a day. Children need plenty of calcium for bone formation and girls in particular need plenty of iron-rich foods such as leafy greens, pulses and lean red meat.

- If you have a family of lean children let them fill up on the carbohydrate foods and low-fat protein foods. (For more information on a healthy diet see chapter 7.) Don't be tempted to fill them up with high-fat foods just because they aren't fat. Eating habits learnt in childhood tend to be the ones we keep for life.

Generally, in Britain children eat far too much saturated fat and too few vegetables and fruit – so please, please do encourage them to eat *well*. That doesn't mean you have to turn them into faddy eaters or health food freaks – you will soon see that the *Fat Attack* plan is neither faddy nor freaky!

Remember, lots of the healthiest foods are also the quickest – fruit, yogurts and bread are just as easy as crisps and biscuits.

Every day on the diet plan

Milk allowance You can have 150ml (1/4 pint) skimmed milk. If you don't want this, have low-fat natural yogurt instead.

Daily treat Every day you can pick one *treat* from the following list.

- 25g (1oz) bar chocolate
- 2 small glasses wine or 1 pint beer or lager
- 1 slice rich fruit cake
- 2 chocolate digestives
- 110g (4oz, two scoops) real dairy ice cream
- A recipe dessert (see pages 138–41)
- 40g (1 1/2oz) Cheddar or Stilton
- 1 packet crisps
- 2 fingers KitKat

- small portion oven chips
- 15g ($^1/_2$oz) butter

Unlimiteds All these foods and drinks are unlimited throughout the 30 days and beyond.

- *Drinks:* Black tea or black coffee (or with milk from allowance); fruit tea; water, mineral water; calorie-free squash; calorie-free fizzy drinks and mixers.
- *Eats:* Any green leaf salad items; pickled onions; yeast extract (Marmite); raw onions; cress; cucumber.
- *Condiments:* Herbs, dried or fresh, all kinds. Spices, dried or fresh, all kinds; chillies; salt and pepper; garlic; Tabasco (chilli sauce); lemon and lime juices; mushroom ketchup; mustard; oyster sauce; soya sauce; vinegar; Worcestershire sauce; oil-free French dressing; tomato purée; artificial sweeteners.

Fruit choices When a 'fruit choice' is mentioned within the plan, choose any of the following that you like. Try to vary your choices as much as possible.

- *One* of the following: apple, slice melon, nectarine, orange, peach, pear, 2 rings pineapple, guava, mango.
- *Two* of the following: apricots, satsumas, clementines, kiwifruit, plums, greengages, figs.
- *Average bowlful* of any of the following, fresh: raspberries, tayberries, blueberries, strawberries, loganberries, fresh fruit salad.
- *Average bowlful* of any of the following, stewed with artificial sweetener: apple, blackberries, blackcurrants, damsons, gooseberries, plums, rhubarb.
- *Small bowlful* of any of the following: cherries, grapes, dessert gooseberries.

Salad choices When 'salad choice' is mentioned within the plan, choose as much as you like in any combination from the following list. Unless a dressing is specified in the plan, you should eat your salad plain or with oil-free French dressing or 2 teaspoons of Kraft Free Choice mayonnaise-style dressing.

- Artichoke hearts
- Bamboo shoots
- Beansprouts of any kind
- Cabbage, raw, red or white, shredded
- Cabbage, red, pickled
- Carrot, raw
- Cauliflower, raw
- Celery
- Chicory
- Chinese leaves
- Courgettes, raw, thinly sliced
- Cucumber
- Endive
- Fennel
- Gherkins
- Herbs, fresh, any kind
- Lettuce, all types and colours
- Mushrooms, raw, sliced
- Mustard and cress
- Olives
- Onions, raw, sliced
- Peppers, raw, any colour
- Radicchio
- Radishes
- Spinach, raw
- Spring onions
- Tomato
- Watercress

Vegetable choices When 'vegetable choices' are mentioned with your evening meal, choose the number of stated portions from the following list. Vegetables should be, in the main, lightly boiled, steamed, microwaved, braised, baked or grilled but occasionally you could stir-fry them using the method on pages 44–5.

- Asparagus
- Leeks

- Aubergine
- Baby corn cobs
- Broad beans
- Broccoli
- Brussels sprouts
- Cabbage, any kind
- Calabrese
- Carrots
- Cauliflower
- Celeriac
- Chinese leaves
- Courgettes
- French beans
- Globe artichokes
- Jerusalem artichokes
- Kale
- Kohlrabi
- Mangetout
- Marrow
- Mixed frozen vegetables
- Mushrooms
- Okra
- Onions
- Peas
- Peppers, any colour
- Runner beans
- Spinach
- Spring greens
- Squash
- Swede
- Sweetcorn
- Tomatoes
- Turnips

Fruit, Salad and vegetables – the ACE choices As I explained at the beginning of this chapter, certain fruit and vegetables are good providers of the ACE anti-oxidant vitamins linked with protection against heart disease and cancer. You should try to get as many of these high-ACE vegetables as possible. Here is a list of the best sources of each of the three ACE vitamins. Bear it in mind when making your daily choices.

Fruits and vegetables containing most vitamin C per portion (especially if raw or very lightly cooked): all citrus fruits, especially oranges; peppers of all colours; broccoli; parsley; Brussels sprouts; all leafy green vegetables; strawberries; blackcurrants; guava; mango; melon; tomatoes. But all fruit and vegetables contain some vitamin C.

Fruits and vegetables containing most beta-carotene per portion: carrots; sweet potatoes*; squash; spinach; broccoli; watercress; dark lettuce leaves; tomatoes; asparagus; peas; dark green cabbage and spring greens; sweetcorn; mangoes; orange-fleshed melons; apricots; peaches; nectarines; oranges.

* Sweet potatoes can be used instead of ordinary potatoes whenever you like – you can bake them, or peel and boil them.

Fruits and vegetables containing most vitamin E: leafy green vegetables; avocados; olives. (Other sources of vitamin E are vegetable oils, nuts, seeds and whole grains including wholemeal bread.)

Portion sizes: One of the first things you will notice on the plan is that I have eliminated weighing and measuring as far as possible. Because this is a reduced-fat diet and not a low-carbohydrate one, you can really eat your fill of the complex carbohydrates, as long as you are sensible. When I mention an 'average' portion of bread, potatoes, rice and other grains, pasta, breakfast cereals and pulses I mean the amount which most people would consider normal and which will satisfy your hunger. For instance, an average bowl of flaked breakfast cereal is around 25g (1oz), an average slice of bread weighs about 40g ($1^1/_2$oz) and an average baked potato is around 225–275g (8–10oz). 'Large' portions will be 25–50 per cent more than this.

'A little low-fat spread' means just enough to moisten your bread or whatever.

Between meals Between meals, if you ever find yourself feeling hungry, eat a piece of fruit or a small piece of bread to fill the gap. Or perhaps you may prefer to have the 'dessert' part of your lunch and/or evening meal (e.g. fruit or yogurt) as a separate snack.

Breakfast Every day you can pick any one of the following seven options. Try to vary your choices at least occasionally. When bread is stated, wholemeal is preferable but white, or any other type of plain bread, is acceptable.

1. *Cereal, bread and fruit*

- Average bowlful plain cereal with 100ml ($3^{1}/_{2}$ fl oz) skimmed milk, extra to allowance (choose from cornflakes, branflakes, Special K, Fruit 'n' Fibre, Puffed Wheat, All Bran, Bran Buds, Rice Krispies or bite-sized Shredded Wheat) *or* 2 Weetabix.
- 1 average slice bread with a little low-fat spread and low-sugar jam or marmalade.
- 1 fruit choice.

2. *Muesli and fruit*

- Average bowlful 'no added sugar' muesli with 100ml (4171 fl oz) skimmed milk extra to allowance.
- 1 fruit choice.

3. *Bread and fruit*

- 2 average slices bread with little low-fat spread and low-sugar jam or marmalade or Marmite.
- 1 fruit choice.

4. *Porridge, bread and fruit*

- Average bowlful porridge made using half water and half skimmed milk with 1 level teaspoon sugar.
- 1 average slice bread with a little low-fat spread and Marmite (optional).
- 1 fruit choice.

5. *Fruit, yogurt and bread*

- Unlimited fresh fruit of choice, chopped if necessary, into 1 small tub low-fat natural yogurt with 1 level teaspoon sugar.
- 1 average slice bread with a little low-fat spread and low-sugar jam or marmalade or Marmite.

6. *Fruit, yogurt and cereal*

- Unlimited fresh fruit of choice, chopped if necessary, into 1 small tub low-fat natural yogurt with 1 level teaspoon sugar and 1 good handful 'no added sugar' muesli *or* 2 good handfuls plain cereal of choice (see list in first option).

7. *Dried fruit, yogurt and cereal*

- 4–5 tablespoons stewed dried fruit of choice (e.g. dried fruit salad or prunes or apricots or peaches) with 1 small tub low-fat natural yogurt and 1 handful 'no added sugar' muesli *or* 2 handfuls plain cereal as before.

(***Note:*** Dried fruit should be stewed without added sugar – it is sweet enough despite the fact that some of the packets tell you to add sugar.)

Lunch There is always a 'packable' option at lunchtimes if needed. There is usually one easy-cook hot option and always at least one cold option.

Lunch is always either a sandwich, something on toast, a recipe soup, a recipe salad or a baked potato with filling.

When a sandwich is specified, you can choose any of these for your bread: any plain bread (try to make full use of the more unusual kinds, such as black rye); one whole pitta, white or wholemeal, split and filled; French bread (an average chunk); 2 petits pains; 1 bagel; 2 small rolls; 1 large bap.

There are always plenty of filling options and don't forget to add plenty of salad – things like lettuce, cress, cucumber and onion are virtually calorie-free but add vitamins and bulk.

When you pick a sandwich option you can, if you wish, arrange the bread, filling (if it is suitable) and salad as a plate meal.

If toast is specified, have up to 2 average slices for an average portion, 3 if you are having large portions.

Evenings There is almost always a choice between a simple, straightforward, minimal-cook meal and a recipe dish – all of which, too, are quite easy. Vegetable accompaniments to your evening meal should never be omitted. You can choose my own recommendations or make your own choices from the lists.

THE 30-DAY PLAN

Day 1

Breakfast
Choose from the options on pages 57–8

Lunch
1 portion Pasta and Tuna Salad (see recipe page 107)
OR
Sandwich with a Group 3 or 4 filling (see page 144)
Fruit choice with either option

Evening
1 portion Greek-Style Spicy Lamb Kebabs (see recipe page 124)
1 portion Tomato Rice (see recipe page 137)
Salad choice – my suggestion is cucumber, green pepper and crisp lettuce
OR
1 average lean lamb steak, grilled
Average serving new potatoes
2 vegetable choices – my suggestion is peas and leeks
Mint sauce and a little fat-free gravy if liked

- Don't forget your daily milk and treats allowance – see pages 52–3.
- Why not make double quantities of Tomato Rice and freeze the rest for another time?

Day 2

Breakfast

Choose from the options on pages 57–8

Lunch

1 average baked potato plus your choice of filling from Group 2, 3 or 4 (see pages 142–3)

OR

Sandwich with your choice of filling from Group 2, 3 or 4 (see pages 143–4)

Fruit choice with either option

Evening

1 portion Hawaiian Pizza (see recipe page 95)

Salad choice – my suggestion is tomato, watercress and lettuce

OR

1 Findus French Bread Pizza, ham and pineapple or ham and mushroom

Salad as above

1 diet fruit fromage frais or yogurt with either option

- Don't forget to have plenty of 'unlimited' salad items with your lunch.
- Remember if you're having a sandwich at lunchtime, you don't have to just stick to sliced brown or white bread – check your choices on pages 143–4.

Day 3

Breakfast

Choose from the options on pages 57–8

Lunch

Toast with a topping of your choice from Group 1, 3 or 4 (see pages 141–3)

OR

Sandwich with a filling from Group 1, 3 or 4 (see pages 143–4)

Fruit choice with either option

Evening

1 portion Chicken Dijon (see recipe page 118)

Average serving boiled potatoes

2 vegetable choices – my suggestion is broccoli and green beans

OR

1 medium chicken breast, skinned, sprinkled with Cajun seasoning and grilled or microwaved

1 portion Salsa (see recipe page 101 or use ready-made)

Average serving long grain rice, boiled

- Remember if you're having toast for lunch you can have two generous slices and a little low-fat spread if necessary.
- A nice change from plain long grain rice is easy-cook long grain and wild rice – it looks pretty, too.

Day 4

Breakfast

Choose from the options on pages 57–8

Lunch

1 portion Lentil and Vegetable Soup (see recipe page 90) with 1 average bread roll

OR

Sandwich with your choice of filling from Group 1, 2, 3 or 4 (see pages 143–4)

Evening

1 portion Pasta with Bacon and Mushrooms (see recipe page 96) topped with 1 level tablespoon grated Parmesan

Salad choice – my suggestion is a mixed leaf green salad

OR

1 pack MenuMaster Healthy Options Lean Beef Lasagne

Salad as above *plus* one large banana

- Home-made soups are really easy and quick to prepare – and if hunger is one of your main problems when you're trying to shed the fat, they are *so* satisfying!
- Convenience meals don't *have* to be high in fat or unhealthy – especially if you add salad or extra vegetables and fruit to your meal.

Day 5

Breakfast

Choose from the options on pages 57–8

Lunch

Toast with a topping of your choice from Group 1, 3 or 4 (see pages141–3)

OR

Sandwich with a filling of your choice from Group 1, 3 or 4 (see pages 143–4)

Fruit choice with either option

Evening

1 portion Barbecued Bean and Sausage Bake (see recipe page 110)

Vegetable choice – my suggestion is spring greens

OR

3 low-fat pork and beef chipolatas, grilled

Average serving mashed potato (made with a little skimmed milk and low-fat spread, or use instant mash)

Average serving baked beans in tomato sauce

1 diet fruit fromage frais or yogurt with either option

Fruit choice with either option

- You can turn almost any traditional British fare into a healthy low-fat meal – like this sausage and mash, for instance!

Day 6

Breakfast

Choose from the options on pages 57–8

Lunch

1 portion Coronation Chicken Salad (see recipe page 104)

1 banana

OR

Sandwich with a filling of your choice from Group 1, 2 or 4 (see pages 143–4)

Fruit choice

Evening

1 portion Salmon Brochettes with Wild Rice (see recipe page 133)

$^1/_2$ portion Salsa (see recipe page 101)

Salad choice – my suggestion is cucumber, spring onions and watercress

OR

1 medium salmon steak or trout or mackerel fillet, grilled or microwaved

Average serving new potatoes

2 vegetable choices – my suggestion is mangetout and broccoli

$^1/_2$ portion Salsa (see recipe page 101) or 1 tablespoon ready-made salsa

- Salmon is quite high in fat but as it is rich in the 'good for you' omega-3 oils do include it in your diet if you can.

Day 7

Breakfast
Choose from the options on pages 57–8

Lunch
1 portion Potato and Watercress Soup (see recipe page 92)
Granary bap with a little low-fat spread
Fruit choice
OR
Sandwich with filling of your choice from Group 3 or 4 (see pages 143–4)
Fruit choice

Evening
1 portion Beef Rendang (see recipe page 113)
Average serving boiled long grain rice
Salad choice – my suggestion is thinly sliced cucumber mixed with thinly sliced red onions and tomatoes
OR
1 portion Spaghetti Bolognese (see recipe page 97)
Salad choice – my suggestion is a mixed green salad
OR
3 slices very lean roast beef or pork
1 medium baked potato
1 portion Roast Vegetables (see recipe page 136) *or* 2–3 vegetable choices – my suggestion is carrots, spring greens and peas
Stock-cube gravy and horseradish or apple sauce

Day 8

Breakfast

Choose from the options on pages 57–8

Lunch

1 portion Egg and Smoked Haddock Salad (see recipe page 105)

OR

Sandwich with a filling of your choice from Group 1, 3 or 4 (see pages 143–4)

Fruit choice with either option

Evening

1 portion Turkey and Noodle Stir-Fry (see recipe page 135)

Fruit choice

OR

1 average turkey steak, grilled

Average serving boiled potatoes or noodles

2 vegetable choices – my suggestion is green beans and courgettes

Stock-cube gravy or 2 tablespoons Tomato Sauce (see recipe page 102)

1 diet fromage frais or fruit yogurt

Fruit choice

- Don't forget your daily treat (for a list of options, see pages 52–3). For instance, today you could have 15g ($^1/_2$oz) butter with your potatoes, a recipe dessert or some wine!

Day 9

Breakfast

Choose from the options on pages 57–8

Lunch

1 portion Pasta and Vegetable Soup (see recipe page 91)
1 granary bap
Fruit choice
OR
Sandwich with filling of your choice from Group 3 or 4 (see page 144)
Fruit choice

Evening

1 portion Balti Chicken with Vegetables and Chapati (see recipe page 109)
Fruit choice
OR
1 filleted breast of chicken, skinned and coated with a paste of low-fat natural yogurt mixed with 1 teaspoon of tandoori powder, grilled
Average serving boiled rice
Salad choice – my suggestion is cucumber and lettuce salad with sliced raw onion
Fruit choice

- If you chose the breast of chicken dinner, today has been a very low-fat day – you could add a little more fat in the form of some real dairy ice cream or a Cheddar portion (see pages 52–3 for complete list of treats) without feeling in the slightest bit guilty!

Day 10

Breakfast

Choose from the options on pages 57–8

Lunch

Toast with a topping of your choice from Group 1, 2 or 4 (see pages 141–3)

OR

Sandwich with your choice of filling from Group 1, 2 or 4 (see pages 143–4)

Fruit choice with either option

Evening

1 portion Piquant Pan-Fried Fish (see recipe page 128)

Average serving new potatoes

2 vegetable choices – my suggestion are broccoli and carrots

OR

1 frozen individual cod or haddock steak in crisp crunch crumb, baked

Potatoes and vegetables as above

1 tablespoon relish or sauce of choice

- Don't forget – keep having plenty of salad items with your lunch or crunch through some crispy carrot or salad mid-afternoon to keep the hunger pangs at bay.

Day 11

Breakfast
Choose from the options on pages 57–8

Lunch
1 portion Mushroom and Bacon Salad (see recipe page 106)
1 granary bap with a little low-fat spread
Fruit choice
OR
Sandwich with your choice of filling from Group 3 or 4 (see page 144)
Fruit choice

Evening
1 portion Beef Goulash (see recipe page 112)
Small serving boiled long grain rice or long grain and wild rice
Vegetable choice – my suggestion is thinly sliced white cabbage – or a large green salad
OR
175 (6oz) lean rump or fillet steak, grilled
1 average baked potato topped with 1/2 portion Salsa (see recipe page 101) *or* low-fat spread or low-fat crème fraîche
2 vegetable choices – my suggestion is peas and broccoli

- A nice glass of red wine would go well with the goulash – and it *is* allowed (see treats list pages 52–3).

Day 12

Breakfast

Choose from the options on pages 57–8

Lunch

1 average baked potato with your choice of topping from Group 1, 2, 3 or 4 (see pages 141–3)

OR

Sandwich with your choice of filling from Group 1, 2, 3 or 4 (see pages 143–4)

Fruit choice with either option

Evening

1 portion Tuna and Pasta Cheese Bake (see recipe page 98)

Salad choice – my suggestion is a large salad of cucumber, endive and watercress

OR

2-egg tuna omelette – beat eggs with a little water and seasoning and make in non-stick pan sprayed with Fry Light. Fill with 50g (2oz) tuna in brine, drained and flaked

Average serving new potatoes *or* bread

Salad choice – my suggestion is a large mixed salad

1 banana

- You could fill the omelette with prawns or extra lean chopped ham instead.

Day 13

Breakfast

Choose from the options on pages 57–8

Lunch

1 portion Prawn and Avocado Salad (see recipe page 108)

Fruit choice

OR

Sandwich with your choice of filling from Group 1, 2, 3 or 4 (see pages 143–4)

Fruit choice

Evening

1 portion Chilli Beef Pizza (see recipe page 94)

Salad choice – my suggestion is a large mixed salad

OR

1 QuarterPounder Beefburger, well grilled, in a burger bun

2 teaspoons burger relish

Salad choice – my suggestion is a large mixed salad

1 banana

- If you choose the burger option in the evening, your treat for the day could be some oven chips to go with it (see treats list on pages 52–3).
- Do remember to vary your choices as much as possible to make quite sure you are getting all the vitamins, minerals and trace elements you need for a healthy diet.

Day 14

Breakfast

Choose from the options on pages 57–58

Lunch

Toast with your choice of topping from Group 1, 3 or 4 (see pages 141–4)

OR

Sandwich with your choice of filling from Group 1, 3 or 4 (see pages 143–4)

Fruit choice with either option

Evening

1 portion lean roast leg of lamb (3–4 slices) *or* 1 lamb steak, grilled

1 portion Roast Vegetables (see recipe page 136) or 2 vegetable choices – my suggestion is carrots and broccoli

1 average baked potato

Stock-cube gravy and mint or redcurrant sauce *or* $^1/_2$ portion Onion Sauce (see recipe page 100)

OR

1 portion Burgundy Beef in Red Wine (see recipe page 115)

Average serving new potatoes

Vegetable choice – my suggestion is broccoli

- If you enjoy roast lamb, do avoid choosing shoulder as it is very, very fatty, whereas leg of lamb is nice and lean. Leg may appear more expensive, but weight for weight there is much more meat on the leg than the shoulder.

Day 15

Breakfast

Choose from the options on pages 57–58

Lunch

Salad – a large mixed salad with a large bap and one small can tuna in brine, drained, plus 2 teaspoons Kraft Free Choice mayonnaise-style dressing

OR

Sandwich with your choice of filling from Group 2, 3 or 4 (see pages 143–4)

Fruit choice with either option

Evening

1 portion Spanish Tortilla (see recipe page 134)

Average portion crusty bread (e.g. French)

Salad choice – my suggestion is a leaf green salad

1 diet fromage frais or fruit yogurt

OR

Large baked potato with a filling of your choice from any group (see pages 141–3)

1 banana and 1 diet fromage frais or fruit yogurt

Salad choice – my suggestion is a large mixed salad

- Don't forget that if you like a big lunch you can add an extra or treat to it from the list on pages 52–3. Another alternative is to have part of your breakfast at breakfast time and save the remainder to have mid-morning as a snack to stave off hunger (see 'breakfast' pages 57–8).

Day 16

Breakfast

Choose from the options on pages 57–8

Lunch

Toast with your choice of topping from Group 2 or 4 (see pages 142–3)

OR

Sandwich with your choice of filling from Group 2 or 4 (see pages 143–4)

Fruit choice with either option

Evening

1 portion Prawn and Mushroom Risotto (see recipe page 130)

Salad choice – my suggestion is a mixed leaf green salad

1 large banana

OR

1 average white or oily fish fillet, grilled or microwaved

Average serving new potatoes

2 vegetable choices – I suggest peas and carrots

2 teaspoons relish of choice

1 large banana

- If you're cooking plain fish, you can liven it up easily. Try sprinkling on lemon juice and black pepper, or a dash of Tabasco hot pepper sauce, or some Lea and Perrins ginger and orange. Or bake in foil with sliced spring onions and fresh herbs such as tarragon or thyme.

Day 17

Breakfast

Choose from the options on pages 57–8

Lunch

1 portion Lentil and Vegetable Soup (see recipe page 90) *or* 1 whole can Heinz Tomato and Lentil or Pea and Ham Soup

1 average roll

OR

Sandwich with your choice of filling from Group 3 or 4 (see page 144)

Evening

1 portion Caribbean Sweet and Sour Pork (see recipe page 116)

Average serving boiled long grain rice or noodles

Salad choice – my suggestion is a large mixed salad

OR

1 average well-trimmed pork steak or chop, grilled

Average serving boiled potatoes

2 vegetable choices – my suggestion is spring greens or red cabbage and peas or sweetcorn

Stock-cube gravy and apple sauce

- If you have a packed lunch, that doesn't stop you enjoying a recipe salad – you can buy an insulated container to pop in your lunchbox.

Day 18

Breakfast

Choose from the options on pages 57–8

Lunch

1 portion Cheese, Ham and Pasta Salad (see recipe on page 103)

OR

Sandwich with your choice of filling from Group 1, 3 or 4 (see pages 143–4)

Fruit choice (with second option only)

Evening

1 portion Barbecue-Style Baked Chicken (see recipe page 111)

1 average baked potato

2 vegetable choices – my suggestion is baby corn cobs and mangetout

OR

1 average chicken breast, plain grilled and skin removed before eating

1 average baked potato or average serving boiled potatoes with 1 teaspoon low-fat spread

2 vegetable choices as above

- If you enjoy doing recipe dishes, get in the habit of cooking some when you have some spare time – most of the evening meals can be frozen.

Day 19

Breakfast

Choose from the options on pages 57–8

Lunch

Toast with a topping of your choice from Group 1, 3 or 4 (see pages 141–3)

OR

Sandwich with a filling of your choice from Group 1, 3 or 4 (see pages 143–4)

Fruit choice with either option

Evening

1 portion Chilli Con Carne (see recipe page 121)

Average serving boiled rice *or* baked potato

Salad choice – my suggestion is a salad of watercress, cucumber, iceberg lettuce and radish

OR

1 average lamb steak, grilled

Average serving boiled potatoes

2 vegetable choices – I suggest broad beans or peas and carrots

Stock-cube gravy and mint or redcurrant sauce

- Chilli cooked the right way and served with plenty of potato or rice is a very healthy meal – so enjoy it!

Day 20

Breakfast

Choose from the options on pages 57–8

Lunch

Average serving three bean salad (ready made and available in most supermarkets)
2 slices smoked turkey
1 average roll with a little low-fat spread

OR

Sandwich with your choice of filling from Group 1, 2 or 4 (see pages 143–4)
Fruit choice with either option

Evening

1 portion Salmon and Broccoli Pancakes (see recipe page 132)
Salad choice – my suggestion is a green salad

OR

Average serving boiled pasta of choice topped with 1 portion Roasted Vegetables (see recipe page 136) and 1 tablespoon crumbled feta cheese or Parmesan

- Penne or pasta spirals go well with the Roasted Vegetables option – mix them in together and top with the cheese for a very pretty dish. If you're in even more of a hurry – top your pasta with Tomato Sauce (see recipe page 102) and Parmesan.
- You can use cannelloni shells instead of the pancakes if you like – buy them ready made from the pasta counter.

Day 21

Breakfast
Choose from the options on pages 57–8

Lunch
1 portion Potato and Watercress Soup (see recipe page 92)
Large bap
OR
Sandwich with your choice of filling from Group 3 or 4 (see page 144)
Fruit choice with either option

Evening
1 portion Beef Stroganoff (see recipe page 114)
Average serving boiled rice or noodles
Salad choice – my suggestion is a mixed salad
OR
Beefburger meal as Day 13

- When ordinary salad leaves are expensive you can make a tasty and pretty salad from finely sliced red cabbage, white cabbage or Chinese leaves and ribbons of carrot.

Day 22

Breakfast
Choose from the options on pages 57–8

Lunch
1 average baked potato with your choice of filling from Group 1, 3 or 4 (see pages 141–3)
OR
Sandwich with your choice of filling from Group 1, 3 or 4 (see pages 143–4)
Fruit choice with either option

Evening
1 portion Chicken Provençal (see recipe page 119)
Average serving boiled rice or potatoes
Vegetable choice – my suggestion is broccoli
OR
Average serving roast chicken (no skin)
Average serving new potatoes baked in their skins, very lightly brushed with oil
2 vegetable choices – my suggestion are broccoli and peas
Stock-cube gravy and 1 tablespoon stuffing

- You can get a lovely crisp modern-style roast potato by leaving skins on, brushing with oil and putting the potatoes in a roasting pan as usual. For even more taste sprinkle with chopped garlic, salt and pepper.

Day 23

Breakfast
Choose from the options on pages 57–8

Lunch
Toast with your choice of topping from Group 2, 3 or 4 (see pages 142–3)
OR
Sandwich with your choice of filling from Group 2, 3 or 4 (see pages 143–4)
Fruit choice with either option

Evening
1 portion Chinese Noodles with Egg and Prawns (see recipe page 122)
Fruit choice
OR
A platter of 1 hard-boiled egg, sliced; 75g (3oz) peeled prawns or tuna in brine, drained; 1 level tablespoon reduced-calorie mayonnaise or 1,000 Island dressing; a selection of salad items – e.g. cucumber, lettuce, cress, tomato, spring onions
1 average roll with a little low-fat spread
Fruit choice and 1 diet fromage frais or fruit yogurt

- If you're choosing the Chinese meal this evening your treat for today could be a Ross frozen Chinese spring roll.

Day 24

Breakfast

Choose from the options on pages 57–8

Lunch

Salad: Mix 1 small can tuna in brine (drained), with 1 tomato (sliced), 2 spring onions (chopped), and half a small can of butter or cannellini beans (drained). Toss all in oil-free French dressing

1 roll or large slice bread

OR

Sandwich with a filling of your choice from Group 1, 3 or 4 (see pages 143–4)

Fruit choice with either option

Evening

1 portion Mediterranean-Style Pork Casserole (see recipe page 125)

1 average baked potato or serving boiled rice

Salad choice – my suggestion is a salad of leaf greens, cress, green pepper and cucumber *or* 1 vegetable choice – my suggestion is spring greens or broccoli

OR

1 average lean pork or turkey steak, grilled

Average serving new potatoes

2 vegetable choices – my suggestion is spring greens and peas

Stock-cube gravy and apple sauce

OR

Any 1 Lean Cuisine for Healthy Appetites plus mixed salad and 1 large banana

Day 25

Breakfast
Choose from the options on pages 57–8

Lunch
1 portion Pasta and Vegetable Soup (see recipe on page 91)
1 large bap with a little low-fat spread
OR
Sandwich with filling of your choice from Groups 2 or 4 (see pages 143–4)
Fruit choice with either option

Evening
1 portion Filo Fish Pie (see recipe page 123)
Average serving baked, mashed or boiled potatoes
Vegetable choice – my suggestion is sweetcorn or courgettes
OR
1 average trout, grilled or microwaved
Potato as above
2 vegetable choices – my suggestion is green beans and sweetcorn

- If you're choosing the trout option today your day's treat could be 25g (1oz) flaked toasted almonds to garnish the trout. Serve with lemon wedges.

Day 26

Breakfast

Choose from the options on pages 57–8

Lunch

1 portion Coronation Chicken Salad (see recipe page 104)

Large banana

OR

Sandwich with filling of your choice from Group 3 or 4 (see page 144)

Fruit choice with second option only

Evening

1 portion Pizza Potatoes (see recipe page 129)

Salad choice – my suggestion is a mixed leaf salad

1 diet fromage frais or fruit yogurt

OR

Large baked potato with filling of your choice from Group 1, 2, 3 or 4 (see pages 141–3)

Salad and dessert as above

OR

Average serving boiled pasta of choice topped with 1 portion Tomato Sauce (see recipe page 102) and 2 level tablespoons Parmesan cheese with salad and dessert as above

- It is a good idea to make up a large batch of tomato sauce and freeze it in single or double portions – it has so many uses.

Day 27

Breakfast
Choose from the options on pages 57–8

Lunch
Toast with your choice of topping from Group 1, 3 or 4 (see pages 141–3)
OR
Sandwich with your choice of filling from Group 1, 3 or 4 (see pages 143–4)
Fruit choice with either option

Evening
1 portion Mexican Chicken Fajitas (see recipe page 126)
Salad choice – my suggestion is iceberg lettuce and cucumber
1 banana
OR
1 chicken portion, baked or grilled, skin removed
Average serving baked, boiled or mashed potatoes
2 vegetable choices – my suggestion is mangetout and green beans
2 teaspoons relish of choice
Stock-cube gravy if liked
1 banana

- Instead of plain grilled chicken and a side relish, you could skin the chicken before grilling and brush on ready-made barbecue sauce, or French mustard for 'devilled chicken'.

Day 28

Breakfast

Choose from the options on pages 57–8

Lunch

1 average baked potato with filling of your choice from Group 3 or 4 (see pages 142–3)

OR

Sandwich with your choice of filling from Group 3 or 4 (see page 144)

Fruit choice with either option

Evening

1 portion Cauliflower and Broccoli Cheese with Ham (see recipe page 117)

1 average slice French bread or large bap

Fruit choice and diet fromage frais or fruit yogurt

OR

MenuMaster Cauliflower Cheese (frozen ready meal)

Bread as above

Salad choice – my suggestion is a tomato, cucumber and onion salad

- Yellow-fleshed sweet potatoes (rather than the white-fleshed variety) make a nice change from ordinary baked potatoes and are rich in beta-carotene. They can be baked in just the same way.

Day 29

Breakfast

Choose from the options on pages 57–8

Lunch

Coleslaw made from shredded white cabbage, grated carrot and onion all mixed together with 1 tablespoon raisins. To dress – beat together 1 tablespoon Kraft Free Choice mayonnaise-style dressing with 1 tablespoon low-fat yogurt, seasoning and lemon juice to taste

2 average slices lean ham or smoked turkey

Large bap or slice French bread with a little low-fat spread

OR

Sandwich with filling of your choice from Group 1, 2, 3 or 4 (see pages 143–4)

Fruit choice with either option

Evening

1 portion Chicken Tikka Masala (see recipe page 120)

Average serving boiled rice

2 teaspoons mango chutney

OR

3–4 slices lean roast chicken (no skin)

1 average baked potato or serving boiled or mashed potato

2 vegetable choices – my suggestion is sweetcorn and courgettes

Stock-cube gravy and 1 tablespoon stuffing

- If you choose the masala dish, today's treat could be an onion bhaji and a poppadum.

Day 30

Breakfast

Choose from the options on pages 57–8

Lunch

1 portion Potato and Watercress soup (see recipe page 92)

1 bap with a little low-fat spread

OR

Sandwich with filling or your choice from Group 3 or 4 (see page 144)

Fruit choice with either option

Evening

1 portion Moussaka (see recipe page 127) *or* Low-fat Lasagne (see recipe page 95)

Small serving new or boiled potatoes

Salad choice – my suggestion is mixed leaves including endive, radish and spring onions

OR

3–4 slices lean roast leg of lamb

1 average baked potato

2 vegetable choices – my suggestion is swede and spring greens

Stock-cube gravy and mint sauce or redcurrant jelly *or* $^1/_2$ portion Onion Sauce (see recipe page 100)

- Don't forget there are some delicious recipe desserts to choose from as your daily treat – see recipes pages 138–141.

CHAPTER 5

The **fat***attack* ***Recipes***

All recipes serve four but quantities can easily be halved to serve two. Although the Fat Attack system does not depend on calorie-counting as such, I have given the calorie and fat counts in case anyone would like them.

SOUPS AND STARTERS

Lentil and Vegetable Soup

(Serves 4; 5.25g fat and 200 calories per portion.)

Here's a hearty soup to satisfy any appetite.

1 tablespoon corn oil
1 large onion, finely chopped
2 level teaspoons mild curry powder
1.1 litre (2 pints) stock
110g (4oz) (dry weight) brown lentils
1 parsnip, diced
2 medium carrots, diced
75g (3oz) swede or turnip, diced
200g (7oz) potato, peeled and diced
2 stalks celery, diced
2 teaspoons tomato purée
Salt and black pepper

Heat the oil in a saucepan and add the onion and curry powder; stir-fry few a few minutes. Add the stock and lentils, bring to simmer and simmer for 30–45 minutes or until lentils are tender. Add rest of ingredients and simmer for a further 30–45 minutes. Check seasoning.

- For a thicker soup you can purée half of it when cooked, then return it to the pan, combining it well with the unpuréed soup.
- You can use beef stock for a very robust soup, or chicken or vegetable stock for a more delicate flavour.
- You can omit the curry powder if you like or substitute a teaspoon of ground cumin.

Pasta and Vegetable Soup

(Serves 4; 1.5g fat and 145 calories per portion.)

This is similar to minestrone but lower in fat and not quite so fiddly to prepare!

2 small courgettes
50g (2oz) green beans
2 medium leeks
2 medium carrots
1 large onion
3 stalks celery
825ml (1½ pints) vegetable or chicken stock
1 × 400g can chopped tomatoes
75g (3oz) (dry weight) small pasta shapes
Salt and black pepper
1 tablespoon tomato purée
1 tablespoon chopped parsley
2 tablespoons grated Parmesan cheese

Chop or slice all the vegetables into small pieces. Place stock, tomatoes and vegetables in a saucepan and simmer, covered, for 30 minutes. Add the pasta, a little salt and pepper, and the tomato purée and simmer for 15 minutes. Check the seasoning and if the soup is too thick add a little water or extra stock.

Serve topped with parsley and cheese.

- You can vary the vegetables almost as you like – e.g., using cabbage instead of courgettes.
- You can also add half a can of cooked haricot or cannellini beans to this soup, which will add 30 calories and no fat per portion.

Potato and Watercress Soup

(Serves 4; 1.7g fat and 150 calories per portion.)

One of the easiest soups imaginable – yet good enough to serve at a dinner party!

540g (1lb) floury potatoes
2 bunches watercress
700ml (1¼ pints) chicken or vegetable stock
275ml (½ pint) semi-skimmed milk
1 small onion, finely chopped
Salt and black pepper

Peel and dice the potatoes into 1 inch (2.5 cm) cubes. Wash and trim the watercress of the thicker stalks and discard any yellow leaves. Reserve a few sprigs. Put all ingredients in saucepan and simmer gently for 20 minutes. Liquidize, return to pan and reheat.

Serve garnished with the reserved watercress.

- You can purchase fresh chilled stocks from most supermarkets – they are usually sold near the fresh chilled soups. Otherwise you could use a good quality stock cube. If you have time you can easily make your own stock by simmering onion, carrots, celery and leeks in water for 30 minutes (for vegetable stock) adding a chicken carcass and giblets (for chicken stock). *No* added fat is needed.

Smoked Trout Pâté

(Serves 4; 4g fat and 100 calories per portion.)

This is good as a starter or a sandwich filling or toast topper.

175g (6oz) smoked trout
75g (3oz) 8 per cent fat natural fromage frais
2 tablespoons Kraft Free Choice mayonnaise-style dressing
2 teaspoons lemon juice
Black pepper

Flake the smoked trout and then blend all the ingredients well together. Check the seasoning and keep in fridge until needed.

PIZZA AND PASTA

Chilli Beef Pizza

(Serves 4; 17g fat and 460 calories per portion.)

Italy meets Mexico for a real filling treat of a supper!

Fry Light spray
225g (8oz) extra lean minced beef
50ml (2 fl oz) beef stock
1 fresh red chilli, de-seeded and finely chopped
Salt and black pepper
1 × 250g jar Italian tomato and mushroom pizza topping
4 spring onions, chopped
2 × 225g deep crust medium pizza bases
50g (2oz) grated mozzarella or half-fat Cheddar
2 tomatoes, sliced
1 small green pepper, de-seeded and cut into thin semi-circles

Spray a non-stick frying pan with Fry Light and heat. Add the minced beef and brown over a medium heat, stirring. When brown, add the stock, chilli and seasoning to pan, stir and simmer for 10 minutes. Add the pizza topping and spring onion, stir well and leave to cool.

Spread the mince topping over the pizza bases evenly. Top with the grated cheese, sliced tomato and green pepper. Bake for 20 minutes at 200°C (400°F, gas mark 6).

- Serve with some green salad for a complete meal.

Hawaiian Pizza

(Serves 4; 11.5g fat and 400 calories per portion.)

1 × 250g jar Italian pizza topping
2 × 225g deep crust medium pizza bases
75g (3oz) Primula Ultra Light low-fat cheese spread
100g (3½oz) extra lean ham, cut into squares
100g (3½oz) pineapple pieces, well drained
50g (2oz) grated mozzarella cheese

Spread the pizza topping evenly over the two bases then put four spoonfuls of the cheese spread on each pizza, spacing them evenly. Arrange the ham squares on the pizzas in between the cheese 'blobs' then scatter the pineapple pieces over. Shake the mozzarella over and bake at 220°C (425°F, gas mark 7) for 15 minutes until cheese is bubbling. Take care not to overcook.

- Primula Ultra Light is the lowest-fat cheese spread that I know of but you can use any 'light' cheese spread and the fat count won't be all that much higher.

Low-fat Lasagne

(Serves 4; 16.25g fat and 435 calories per portion.)

1 (4-serving) quantity of Bolognese sauce adapted as below
1 (4-serving) quantity Cheese Sauce (see recipe page 99)
8 sheets 'no precook' lasagne
1 tablespoon grated Parmesan cheese

Make a Bolognese sauce following the recipe on page 97 – *but* use 275g (10oz) lean minced beef instead of 325g (12oz) and use an extra 50ml (2 fl oz) beef stock (175ml,

6 fl oz, in all). You need the extra moist mixture because the lasagne sheets will soak this up during cooking.

While the meat sauce is cooking, make the cheese sauce.

When both are ready, spoon half the meat sauce into the base of a square lasagne dish and top with half the lasagne sheets. Spoon in the rest of the meat sauce and then cover with the remaining lasagne. Pour the cheese sauce carefully over the top and sprinkle the Parmesan over. Bake at 200°C (400°F, gas mark 6) for 30 minutes or until lasagne is bubbling and top is golden.

Pasta with Bacon and Mushrooms

(Serves 4; 11.5g fat and 475 calories per portion.)

1 tablespoon olive oil
1 large onion, finely chopped
6 slices extra lean, trimmed back bacon, cut crosswise into strips
1 × 400g can chopped tomatoes
1 clove garlic, chopped (optional)
225g (8oz) small mushrooms, sliced
100ml (3½ fl oz) Passata
1½ tablespoons chopped basil
Salt and black pepper
325g (12oz) (dry weight) penne pasta or spirals
2 tablespoons low-fat crème fraîche
8 stoned black olives, halved
4 dried tomatoes, chopped

Heat the oil in a large non-stick frying pan and stir-fry the onion until soft. Stir in the bacon and cook until crisp. Add the canned tomatoes, garlic, mushrooms and Passata, half the basil, seasoning, and simmer for 10 minutes.

Meanwhile, cook the pasta in plenty of boiling salted water until just tender and drain.

Add the crème fraîche to the sauce and stir in.

Serve over the pasta, topped with the olives and dried tomatoes and the rest of the basil.

- Penne pasta are thick quills. Try tricolour pasta for a change. Macaroni also works well with this sauce.

Spaghetti Bolognese

(Serves 4; 9.5g fat and 510 calories per portion.)

This Bolognese sauce is just as rich and tasty as the classic high-fat version.

1 tablespoon olive oil
1 large onion, finely chopped
2 sticks celery, chopped
325g (12oz) extra lean minced beef
1 × 400g tin chopped tomatoes
1 medium carrot, finely chopped
110g (4oz) mushrooms, chopped
1 cup beef stock from cube
1 tablespoon tomato purée
1 clove garlic, crushed (optional)
Dash of red or dry white wine (optional)
2 teaspoons dried Mediterranean herb mix
Salt and black pepper to taste
300g (11oz) (dry weight) durum wheat spaghetti

Heat the oil in large non-stick pan and stir-fry the onion and celery for 4 minutes. Add the beef and stir again until browned. Add the rest of the sauce ingredients, mix well and simmer for a minimum of 30 minutes (longer is better). Add extra beef stock or water if the sauce looks a little dry.

Meanwhile, boil the spaghetti in plenty of salted water until just tender, drain, and serve with the sauce.

- Ready-grated Parmesan cheese adds only around 2g of extra fat per rounded tablespoon and 30 calories.

Tuna and Pasta Cheese Bake

(Serves 4; 11g fat and 475 calories per portion.)

Everyone will love this dish – it takes a while but is extremely easy to make.

1 tablespoon olive oil
1 large onion, chopped
2 medium courgettes, sliced into rounds
1 red pepper, de-seeded and chopped
1 green pepper, de-seeded and chopped
1 clove garlic, chopped (optional)
175g (6oz) (dry weight) pasta shells or macaroni
2 × 184g cans tuna in brine, drained
1 × 400g can chopped tomatoes
100ml (3½ fl oz) (approximately) Passata
Salt and black pepper
1 teaspoon dried oregano
1 (4-serving) quantity Cheese Sauce (see recipe page 99)
50g (2oz) brown breadcrumbs
25g (1oz) grated mozzarella or half-fat Cheddar cheese

Heat the oil in a large non-stick frying pan and stir-fry the onion until slightly softened. Add the courgettes, peppers and garlic and stir-fry for 5 minutes until everything is taking on a golden hint.

Meanwhile, cook the pasta in plenty of salted boiling water until just tender; drain.

Add the pasta, tuna, canned tomatoes and Passata to the frying pan with the seasoning and oregano. You should have a mixture that is slightly drier than a sauce but not too dry. If it does seem too dry, add some more Passata.

Transfer this mixture to a shallow ovenproof dish. Pour the cheese sauce evenly over the top. Mix the breadcrumbs with the cheese and sprinkle over. Bake at 190°C (375°F, gas mark 5) for 30 minutes or until the top is bubbling and golden.

- This is ideal served with a green salad.
- The basic mixture without the pasta or cheese sauce also makes a tasty sauce for a plate of tagliatelle if you want something quicker. This would be around 150 calories per portion with 3.75g fat per portion.

SAUCES AND SALADS

Cheese Sauce

(Serves 4; 5.25g fat and 122 calories per portion.)

This version contains less than half the fat and calories of a normal cheese sauce but it's hard to tell the difference.

25g (1oz) low-fat spread
25g (1oz) (1 rounded tablespoon) plain flour
400ml (14 fl oz) skimmed milk
75g (3oz) grated half-fat Cheddar
Salt and white pepper

Melt the low-fat spread in a small non-stick saucepan. Add the flour and stir until the flour and fat are thoroughly mixed together. Cook gently for 2 minutes, stirring frequently. Slowly add the milk to the pan, stirring all the time. When all the milk is added let the sauce simmer for a minute or two, by which time it should be a good pouring consistency. Add the cheese, stir; season to taste.

- Avoid lumpy sauce: make sure the milk isn't too cold before it goes into the saucepan. Make sure to cook the flour and fat roux for a while before adding the milk. Stir the sauce well every time you add some more milk.
- Use this sauce whenever you would use a cheese sauce – e.g. for cauliflower cheese, macaroni cheese, fish in cheese sauce, as well as for recipes in this book such as Tuna and Pasta Cheese Bake (see page 98).

Onion Sauce

(Serves 4; 2.5g fat and 76 calories per portion.)

1 medium onion, very thinly sliced
110ml (4 fl oz) chicken or vegetable stock from cube, or water
25g (1oz) low-fat spread
25g (1oz) plain flour
275ml ($^1/_2$ pint) skimmed milk
Salt and white pepper to taste

Simmer the onion in the stock (or water) in a small pan for 20 minutes or until the onion is soft. Set the pan to one side. Melt the low-fat spread in a small non-stick pan and add the flour; stir for a minute over a gentle heat. Slowly add the onion stock to the pan, stirring all the time, then add the milk in two or three stages, again stirring. The sauce will thicken, at which stage let it simmer for a minute or two, adding salt and pepper to taste.

- Onion sauce is a delicious, lower-fat alternative to cheese sauce; especially good with roast or grilled lamb and pleasant, too, with gammon steak.

Salsa

(Serves 4–8; 1.8 or 3.75 g fat and 24 or 48 calories per portion.)

Salsa perks up any grilled meat, poultry or fish and can also be used as an instant topping for pasta.

450g (1lb) fresh tomatoes
3 spring onions
1 clove garlic
1 tablespoon olive oil
1 tablespoon fresh basil, chopped
½ green chilli, de-seeded and finely chopped
Salt and black pepper

Peel the tomatoes by making a cross in the top of each and immersing in boiling water for 30 seconds – the skins will then come off easily. In a bowl, chop the tomatoes. Chop the spring onions and add them to the bowl. Very finely chop the garlic and add it with the oil, basil, chilli and seasoning to the bowl and combine thoroughly. Chill for a few hours if possible before serving.

- You can add other ingredients to a salsa if you like – finely chopped green peppers or cucumber, for instance.

Tomato Sauce

(Serves 4; 4g fat and 65 calories per portion.)

A good basic sauce with dozens of uses. Make a big batch and freeze the surplus.

1 tablespoon olive oil
1 onion, finely chopped
25ml (1 fl oz) white wine
1 × 400g can chopped tomatoes
1 tablespoon tomato purée
Dash Worcestershire sauce
1 clove garlic, crushed (optional)
1 level teaspoon brown sugar
1 level teaspoon dried basil
Salt and black pepper

Heat the oil in a saucepan and over a medium heat cook the onion until soft. Add the remaining ingredients and stir well. Simmer, uncovered, for about 30 minutes until the sauce has darkened and thickened. Check for seasoning.

- Some simple additions can vary the sauce: add basil and Parmesan for a pasta topping; add some chopped chilli for a Mexican sauce.

Cheese, Ham and Pasta Salad

(Serves 4; 9.5g fat and 365 calories per portion.)

This incredibly cheesy-tasting salad will delight every cheese-lover's palate.

175g (6oz) (raw weight) tricolour pasta spirals
100g ($3^1/_2$oz) very low-fat cheese spread
50 ml (2 fl oz) natural Bio yogurt
50 ml (2 fl oz) Kraft Free Choice 1,000 Island-style dressing
1 teaspoon Dijon mustard
Salt and black pepper
100g ($3^1/_2$oz) Edam or feta cheese, cut into small cubes
50g (2oz) sultanas or black grapes, de-pipped and halved
100g ($3^1/_2$oz) extra lean ham, cut into bite-sized squares
2 sticks celery, diced
1 red apple

Cook the pasta in boiling salted water until just tender – about 10 minutes. Drain and tip into serving bowl; tip in the cheese spread and mix to combine.

Meanwhile, in a small bowl beat the yogurt with the 1,000 Island, mustard and a little seasoning. Tip the cheese, sultanas (or grapes), ham and celery into this, and finally chop the apple and add to the dressing.

Tip the dressing mixture over the pasta and mix well.

- You can use half-fat Cheddar instead of Edam or feta if you like.
- If you use grapes rather than sultanas the calorie count will be lower.

Coronation Chicken Salad

(Serves 4; 5.5g fat and 265 calories per portion.)

A rich and satisfying salad that tastes wicked – but isn't.

325g (12oz) new potatoes
50g (2oz) 'no need to soak' dried apricots
2 sticks celery
Iceberg lettuce leaves
10 tablespoons Kraft Free Choice mayonnaise-style dressing
1 teaspoon medium curry powder or to taste
2 teaspoons lemon juice
2 teaspoons reduced-sugar apricot jam
Salt and black pepper
1 red apple
325g (12oz) cooked chicken (meat only), cubed
Fresh coriander leaves or parsley, chopped
Pinch paprika

Boil the potatoes, leave to cool and chop into bite-sized chunks. Chop apricots and celery. Line a serving dish (or dishes) with iceberg lettuce leaves. In a bowl, mix the dressing with the curry powder, lemon juice, jam and seasoning. Finally, chop the apple and combine all ingredients then tip on the lettuce leaves. Sprinkle with coriander (or parsley) and paprika.

Egg and Smoked Haddock Salad

(Serves 4; 5.5g fat and 290 calories per portion.)

450g (1lb) smoked haddock fillets
100g (3½oz) (dry weight) vegetable rice
250ml (9 fl oz) vegetable stock
3 tomatoes, chopped
4 spring onions, chopped
4 stoned black olives, quartered
110g (4oz) cooked green beans, halved
6 tablespoons oil-free French dressing mixed with 1 good teaspoon dry mustard
Salt
Lettuce leaves
3 eggs, hard boiled

Make sure there is no skin on the haddock, then poach in a little water for 10 minutes.

Boil the vegetable rice in the stock until rice is tender and all stock absorbed and leave to cool.

When the haddock is cool, gently flake and combine with all the rest of the ingredients except eggs and lettuce.

Arrange the lettuce on the serving dish and pile the rice mixture on top. Cut the eggs into quarters and use for garnish.

Mushroom and Bacon Salad

(Serves 4; 8.5g fat and 155 calories per portion.)

1 tablespoon groundnut or corn oil
650g (1½ lb) mixed mushrooms
(e.g. brown caps and shii-take)
2 tablespoons oil-free French dressing
2 tablespoons light soya sauce
100g (3½ oz) Chinese leaves, sliced
4 lollo rosso leaves, torn
8 baby sweetcorn, lightly boiled and cut into 3 pieces each
225g (8oz) lean back bacon, grilled and chopped
1 bunch watercress, divided

Heat the oil in a non-stick frying pan and stir-fry the mushrooms for 2 minutes over a high heat – making sure to stir all the time. Remove pan from heat and leave.

Combine the dressing and soya sauce. Arrange the salad leaves in a serving bowl. Toss the dressing into the frying pan with the baby corn and bacon and mix with the mushrooms. Transfer the mushroom salad into the serving bowl and garnish with the watercress.

Serve slightly warm.

- This salad should always be eaten with a high-carbohydrate accompaniment, such as crusty bread, unless you are serving it as a starter.

Pasta and Tuna Salad

(Serves 4; 1g fat and 305 calories per portion.)

110g (4oz) (dry weight) pasta shapes of choice
3 tablespoons low-fat natural yogurt
3 tablespoons Kraft Free Choice
mayonnaise-style dressing
1 teaspoon lemon juice
Pinch dry mustard
Pinch sugar
50ml (2 fl oz) skimmed milk
Salt and black pepper
Lettuce leaves
1 red apple
2 × 200g cans tuna in brine, drained
1 × 400g can cannellini beans, drained
1 inch (2.5 cm) cucumber, chopped
1 stick celery, chopped
50g (2oz) cooked green beans,
cut into 1 inch (2.5 cm) pieces
2 tablespoons chopped parsley

Boil the pasta in salted water until just cooked, drain and cool.

Combine the dressing ingredients and check the seasoning. Line serving bowl with lettuce leaves. Chop the apple and combine all the ingredients except the parsley.

Place the salad on the lettuce leaves, garnish with parsley.

Prawn and Avocado Salad

(Serves 4; 10g fat and 310 calories per portion.)

Avocado is a high-fat fruit but rich in mono-unsaturates and vitamin E.

140g (5oz) (raw weight) long grain rice
8 large lettuce leaves
275g (10oz) peeled prawns
4 canned artichoke hearts, quartered
1 small yellow pepper, de-seeded and chopped
Approximately 4 tablespoons oil-free French dressing mixed with 1 level teaspoon dry mustard or curry powder
1 large, ripe avocado (around 175g or 6oz)

Boil the rice in 325ml (12 fl oz) salted water in a lidded saucepan until all water is absorbed and rice is tender (add extra water if rice dries out before it is tender).

Tear lettuce leaves and arrange them in serving dish (or dishes). Turn cooked rice into a bowl and leave to cool a little, then add the prawns, artichokes, pepper and dressing. Lastly peel, stone and chop the avocado and add to the dish. Toss well.

Serve on top of the lettuce leaves.

- You can add saffron or turmeric powder to the rice cooking water if you like 'yellow rice' – saffron adds a delicious delicate flavour; turmeric a more pungent one.
- You can use lean cooked chicken or ham instead of the prawns in this recipe but add 2g fat and 15 calories per portion extra.

MAIN MEALS AND VEGETABLES

Balti Chicken with Vegetables and Chapati

(Serves 4; 14g fat and 470 calories per portion.)

Balti curries are much quicker to cook than traditional curries. Here's a quick and easy way to enliven a jar of ready-made Balti sauce for an even quicker version.

1 tablespoon corn oil
325g (12oz) lean boneless chicken, skinned and cut into strips
225g (8oz) cauliflower, cut into small florets and parboiled for 2 minutes
225g (8oz) green beans, cut into two
225g (8oz) aubergine, cut into small cubes and parboiled for 2 minutes
2 medium tomatoes, quartered
1 × 400g jar Balti Shahee sauce
4 chapatis

Heat the oil in a large non-stick frying pan and stir-fry the chicken for a few minutes until turning golden. Add all the vegetables and stir-fry for 5 minutes. Add Balti sauce, stir and then simmer for 10 minutes.

Heat the chapatis in a non-stick pan with no oil until each side is blistered and serve with the curry.

- Rice can be served instead of the chapatis for an even lower-fat meal.
- Hungry people can have chapatis and rice – add 20 extra calories and no fat for each tablespoon of cooked rice.

Barbecued Bean and Sausage Bake

(Serves 4; 10.5g fat and 435 calories per portion.)

This is real comfort food and makes an interesting change from basic 'bangers and mash'.

450g (1lb) old potatoes
1 × 420g can baked beans in tomato sauce
1 × 200g can red kidney beans, drained
6 large low-fat pork sausages
1 × 205g jar barbecue marinade
4 tablespoons Passata
2 tablespoons grated Parmesan cheese

Peel and boil the potatoes until barely cooked, cool and slice into rounds about 1/4 inch (0.5 cm) thick.

Meanwhile, grill the sausages and cut into 1/2 inch (1cm) chunks.

In an ovenproof dish, mix the baked beans, kidney beans, sausages and marinade. Top with potato slices and drizzle the Passata over them. Sprinkle on the Parmesan and bake at 200°C (400°F, gas mark 6) for 30 minutes until the top is golden.

- The bake should be served with some broccoli or a green salad.

Barbecue-Style Baked Chicken

(Serves 4; 5g fat and 185 calories per portion.)

This makes an easy change from plain grilled chicken.

3 tablespoons tomato purée
2 tablespoons runny honey
2 tablespoons Worcestershire sauce
1 teaspoon ground cumin
2 teaspoons lemon or lime juice
4 medium chicken portions, skin removed
Sprigs of fresh rosemary or thyme (optional)

In a small bowl, mix all the coating ingredients together and brush on to the chicken pieces. If possible, leave to marinate for an hour or two. Place on a baking sheet with the fresh herbs scattered around and bake at 190°C (375°F, gas mark 5) for 3 minutes.

If there is any marinade mixture left, baste the chicken with it halfway through cooking time.

- You can of course barbecue or grill the chicken pieces using a medium heat.
- This is nice served with baked potatoes and baby corn cobs and mangetout, or with rice, chutney and salad.

Beef Goulash

(Serves 4; 14g fat and 425 calories per portion.)

This dish has real man appeal – but I never found a woman or teenager who didn't love it too!

1 tablespoon corn oil
2 medium onions, sliced
450g (1lb) lean braising steak, cut into cubes
2 tablespoons Hungarian paprika
Pinch ground chilli
1 teaspoon ground caraway seeds
1 medium red pepper, de-seeded and sliced
275ml (1/2 pint) beef stock
1 @ 400g can tomatoes
1 glass red wine
Salt and black pepper
550g (1 1/4 lb) potatoes
50g (2oz) low-fat crème fraîche or Greek yogurt
Chopped parsley to garnish

Heat half the oil in a non-stick flameproof pan and fry the onion until soft and golden. Remove onion with a slatted spatula and reserve. Add other half of the oil to the pan and brown the beef in four batches over a fairly high heat. Add spices and red pepper and stir for half a minute. Add stock, tomatoes, wine and seasoning and return onions to pan. Stir, bring to simmer, and cover. Allow to simmer gently for 1 1/2 hours. Peel the potatoes and cut them into 1 1/2 inch (4cm) chunks, and when the 1 1/2 hours is up add them to the pan. Simmer for a further 30 minutes or until meat and potatoes are tender.

Serve the goulash with a blob of crème fraîche or yogurt for everyone, garnished with the parsley.

- The goulash is best served with a green salad or broccoli or green beans. Very hungry people can add some boiled rice.
- Crème fraîche is a type of French soured cream, with a low-fat version widely available.

Beef Rendang

(Serves 4; 20g fat and 320 calories per portion.)

This Malaysian curry is a truly delicious change from ordinary beef curry – and just as easy.

Few sprays of Fry Light
2 teaspoons groundnut or corn oil
450g (1lb) lean braising steak, cut into cubes
2 medium red onions, cut into wedges
2 medium red peppers, de-seeded and sliced
1 × 35g pack Rendang spices
1 heaped tablespoon tomato purée
1 × 400ml can coconut milk
½ stick lemon grass (optional)
juice of 1 lime
1 small green chilli, de-seeded
and chopped (optional)
Salt and black pepper

Heat a large non-stick lidded frying pan or flameproof casserole and spray with Fry Light to coat evenly. Add the oil. When hot, stir-fry the beef, onion and peppers until meat is brown and vegetables slightly softened and turning golden.

Add the Rendang spices and stir for half a minute, then add remaining ingredients. Bring to simmer, cover and cook for 1 hour or until steak is tender. Check occasionally that the simmer is gentle.

Note: Rendang spices do contain lemon grass and chilli but adding them fresh if available gives the curry even more aroma. Omit the fresh chilli if you prefer your curry medium hot rather than hot.

- Leftover roast beef can be used in this recipe – in which case you can reduce the cooking time to 30 minutes.
- Most supermarkets stock packs of Rendang spices – the most widely available brand name is 'Singapore Spices by Gold Mountain Gourmet'.

Beef Stroganoff

(Serves 4; 16.5g fat and 285 calories per portion.)

In this version, the gloriously rich taste belies the relatively low fat content.

15g (1/2oz) butter
325g (12oz) lean steak, cut into thin strips
2 teaspoons corn oil
1 medium onion, finely chopped
325g (12oz) small mushrooms, halved
2 level teaspoons paprika
1 tablespoon brandy or dry sherry
225ml (8 fl oz) beef stock
1 teaspoon lemon juice
150ml (1/4 pint) low-fat crème fraîche
Salt and black pepper

Heat the butter in a non-stick frying pan and add the steak. Turn it after 1 minute and cook for a further minute; remove. Add the oil to the pan and stir-fry the onion until soft. Add the mushrooms and paprika and stir; add the brandy or sherry and bubble. Add the stock and simmer for a few minutes. Return the beef to the pan and simmer for two more minutes.

Remove pan from heat, add lemon juice and crème fraîche and stir. Season to taste. Serve straight away.

- Use the best-quality steak you can afford – fillet is best, but rump will be fine. You can also make stroganoff using lean fillet of pork.
- Stroganoff is good with rice or noodles and a plain green salad.

Burgundy Beef in Red Wine

(Serves 4; 9g fat and 360 calories per portion.)

Simple to make but impressive enough to give to guests.

2 teaspoons corn oil
450g (1lb) lean cut braising steak, cubed
20 small onions, peeled
50g (2oz) lean bacon, diced
1 × 400g can haricot beans, drained
175g (6oz) carrots, sliced
225g (8oz) button mushrooms
200g (7oz, half a large can) tomatoes
150ml (1/4 pint) beef stock
275ml (1/2 pint) red wine
1 level tablespoon chopped fresh thyme
(or 1 teaspoon dried)
1 large clove garlic, crushed (optional)
1 bay leaf
Salt and black pepper
2 teaspoons cornflour mixed with a little cold water

Brush a non-stick frying pan with the oil and, over a medium to high heat, brown the beef. Remove meat and place in casserole dish. Add the onions and bacon to the frying pan and stir-fry until the onion is softened and bacon golden. Transfer to the casserole. Add the rest of the ingredients except the cornflour, stir and cook, covered, at 150°C (300°F, gas mark 2) for 2 hours.

Add the cornflour, stir well and cook for a further 15 minutes.

Caribbean Sweet and Sour Pork

(Serves 4; 17g fat and 306 calories per portion.)

A nice variation on Chinese sweet and sour, with a creamy yet tangy flavour.

1 tablespoon corn oil
1 medium onion, chopped
1 large red pepper, de-seeded and diced
450g (1lb) lean pork fillet, cubed
1 teaspoon allspice
150g (5½oz) pineapple pieces
25g (1oz) creamed coconut
Juice of 1 lime
1 tablespoon pineapple juice
100ml (3½ fl oz) sweet and sour sauce from a jar (e.g. Sharwoods)
50ml (2 fl oz) water

Heat the oil in a flameproof casserole and stir-fry the onion and pepper over a medium heat for a few minutes. Add pork and fry until edges are golden. Add rest of ingredients and stir. Cover and simmer for 20 minutes.

Cauliflower and Broccoli Cheese with Ham

(Serves 4; 10g fat and 260 calories per portion.)

This is nicer and prettier than plain old cauliflower cheese and makes a more substantial meal.

1 medium cauliflower, broken into large florets
1 medium head broccoli, broken into large florets
225g (8oz) extra lean ham, cut into strips
1 (4-serving) quantity Cheese Sauce
(see recipe page 99)
2 tomatoes, sliced
2 tablespoons Parmesan cheese
2 tablespoons grated reduced-fat Cheddar

Boil the cauliflower and broccoli in salted water until lightly cooked; drain. Arrange in a shallow baking dish with the ham slices. Make the cheese sauce and pour over the vegetables. Arrange the tomato slices round the edge of the dish and sprinkle the two cheeses over the whole thing.

Grill under a medium heat until the top is bubbling and golden.

- The best accompaniment to this is some crusty French bread.

Chicken Dijon

(Serves 4; 11g fat and 290 calories per portion.)

All my family love this dish – and so do I, because it looks and tastes like a real gourmet dish but takes no special skill to make.

1 tablespoon corn oil
4 × 125g (4½oz) boneless chicken breasts, skinned
8 shallots or other small onions, peeled
2 carrots, sliced
2 leeks, sliced
1 tablespoon flour
250ml (9 fl oz) semi-skimmed milk
125ml (4½ fl oz) chicken stock
125ml (4½ fl oz) dry white wine
1 teaspoon fresh thyme
Salt and black pepper
2 tablespoons Dijon mustard
Chopped chives to garnish

Heat the oil in a large flameproof casserole and lightly brown the chicken pieces; remove. Add the vegetables and stir-fry for a minute or two. Add the flour and stir until well blended. Add the milk, stock and wine, and bring to simmer, stirring all the time. Return the chicken to the pan with the thyme and seasoning. Simmer for 30 minutes, covered.

Add the mustard and stir well before serving, garnished with the chives.

- You can omit the wine if you like and use chicken stock instead to make up the liquid.
- Don't use English mustard (dry or made up) in this dish – it will be far too hot.

Chicken Provençal

(Serves 4; 13.5g fat and 280 calories per portion.)

I've added plenty of vegetables to make this Mediterranean chicken casserole incredibly filling.

1 medium aubergine
2 tablespoons olive oil
4 chicken breast fillets, each skinned and cut diagonally into two
1 large onion, sliced
2 green peppers, de-seeded and sliced
1 level tablespoon plain flour
1 × 400g can chopped tomatoes
150ml (1/4 pint) chicken stock
150ml (1/4 pint) dry white wine
1 clove garlic, crushed
110g (4oz) button mushrooms
1 tablespoon tomato purée
1 level teaspoon dried oregano
Salt and black pepper
8 stoned black olives (optional)

Brush the aubergine slices with half the oil and grill (or dry-fry in a non-stick frying pan) for 5 minutes each side until golden.

Meanwhile, heat the rest of the oil in a large flameproof casserole, add the chicken, onion and green peppers, and stir-fry for 4–5 minutes until everything is taking on a golden tinge. Add the flour and stir. Add the aubergine and rest of ingredients, except the olives, and either simmer on the hob for 45 minutes or cook in the oven at 180°C (350°F, gas mark 4) for same length of time.

Add the olives and serve.

Chicken Tikka Masala

(Serves 4; 12g fat and 285 calories per portion.)

Everyone's favourite – but incredibly fattening – Indian meal is transformed here into something equally delicious that you can eat without guilt! And it is so easy it has to be my number one favourite supper.

2 teaspoons corn oil
4 boneless chicken breasts, skinned and each cut into six pieces
2 tablespoons tikka powder (not paste) or to taste
200ml (7 fl oz) full-fat Greek yogurt
Juice of 1 lime
Salt and black pepper
8 teaspoons mango chutney

Heat the oil in a heavy flameproof casserole and gently stir-fry the chicken pieces until they have turned white and are just tinged golden at the edges. Turn the heat down and add the tikka powder; stir. Add the yogurt and stir again. Put the lid on and simmer very gently for about 15 minutes, checking from time to time that the simmer is low.

Add the lime juice and a little seasoning before serving with the mango chutney.

- All you need with this dish is plenty of plain boiled Basmati – or easy cook Basmati – and wild rice and a cucumber salad.
- Don't use low-fat yogurt in this dish – it will separate.

Chilli Con Carne

(Serves 4; 10g fat and 290 calories per portion.)

This is the perfect meal to give to anyone who can't believe they can cut their fat intake and retain all the flavour and filling power in their favourite dishes!

1 tablespoon corn oil
1 large onion, finely chopped
1 stick celery, finely chopped
1 large green pepper, de-seeded and chopped fairly small
325g (12oz) lean minced beef
300ml (1/2 pint) beef stock
2 tablespoons tomato purée
2 teaspoons Worcestershire sauce
1 large fresh green chilli, de-seeded and chopped or chilli powder to taste
1 × 400g can kidney beans, drained and rinsed
1 × 400g can chopped tomatoes
Salt and black pepper

Heat the oil in a large non-stick pan and stir-fry the onion, celery and pepper until soft. Add the beef and stir to brown it. Add the rest of the ingredients, stir and simmer for 30 minutes or more. Check hotness of chilli halfway through – add more chilli as required.

- Serve with plain boiled rice or baked potato and green salad.

Chinese Noodles with Egg and Prawns

(Serves 4; 15.5g fat and 475 calories per portion.)

Chinese food doesn't have to be fatty – and fattening.

250g (9oz) (dry weight) medium egg noodles
1 tablespoon sesame or groundnut oil
4 large or 8 small spring onions, chopped
1 clove garlic, chopped (optional)
1 small lump fresh ginger
110g (4oz) mushrooms – preferably shii-take, sliced
50g (2oz) canned bamboo shoots, sliced
125g (4½oz) fresh beansprouts
25g (1oz) canned water chestnuts, sliced
40g (1½oz) shelled raw unsalted cashew nuts
1 tablespoon dry sherry
Dash soya sauce
Pinch sugar
225g (8oz) peeled prawns
3 size 3 eggs, beaten

Bring a pan of water to the boil and add the noodles; remove from heat and leave for 6 minutes or according to instructions.

Meanwhile, heat the oil in a large non-stick frying pan or wok and stir in the onion, garlic and ginger. Stir half a minute. Add all the vegetables and stir for a minute. Add the nuts, sherry, soya sauce, sugar, and stir. Add prawns and eggs and stir to scramble.

Serve the drained noodles and serve the stir-fry on the noodles as soon as the egg is set.

Filo Fish Pie

(Serves 4; 9g fat and 335 calories per portion.)

Filo is much easier to use than many people think – and gives a much prettier, crunchier top than ordinary pastry.

50g (2oz) (dry weight) split peas
1 large leek, cut into thin rounds
2 medium carrots, cut into thin rounds
110g (4oz) broccoli, cut into small florets
500g (1lb 2oz) white fillet of fish (e.g. cod or haddock)
25g (1oz) low-fat spread
25g (1oz) plain flour
275ml (1/2 pint) stock (see below)
275ml (1/2 pint) skimmed milk
Salt and black pepper
6 square sheets filo pastry (about 4oz, 100g)
1 tablespoon olive oil

Boil the split peas in unsalted water for 30–45 minutes until tender; drain. Parboil the leek and carrot in 275ml (1/2 pint) very lightly salted water until nearly cooked; drain, retaining the cooking water. Parboil the broccoli in a little water and drain (don't keep this water).

Now poach the fish in the retained vegetable water in a pan for a few minutes until barely cooked. Drain, retaining the poaching water.

Flake the fish into the base of a shallow square baking dish and arrange the vegetables and peas in the dish. Strain the vegetable and fish stock through a sieve into a jug. Heat the low-fat spread in a small saucepan and add the flour, stirring, for 1 minute. Gradually add the stock, stirring all the time over a medium heat, then add the milk and cook gently, stirring, until you have a smooth pouring sauce. Season to taste. Pour the sauce evenly over the fish and vegetables.

Brush each filo sheet in turn with a little of the oil and use to cover the fish, slightly concertina-ing each sheet to look pretty. Bake at 190°C (375°F, gas mark 5) for 20 minutes or until the top is golden.

- You can use the basic pie mixture with a mashed potato topping for a change for roughly the same fat and calorie content. Or try a layer of breadcrumbs mixed with 50g (2oz) low-fat grated Cheddar cheese for the same count again.

Greek-Style Spicy Lamb Kebabs

(Serves 4; 15.25g fat and 226 calories per portion.)

450g (1lb) lean lamb fillet, cut into bite-sized cubes
100g (3½oz) low-fat Greek yogurt (e.g. Total)
1 small onion, puréed in blender or very finely chopped
1 garlic clove, crushed (optional)
2 bay leaves
1 tablespoon chopped mint
2 teaspoons paprika
2 teaspoons ground cumin
2 teaspoons ground coriander
1 tablespoon olive oil
Salt and black pepper
1 large red pepper, cut into squares the same size as the lamb

In a bowl, blend all the ingredients except the red pepper and leave for several hours (if possible) to marinate, covered, in a cool place.

When you are ready to cook the kebabs, thread the marinaded lamb pieces on to 4 large kebab sticks with the red pepper pieces. Place on grill pan and brush with a little more of the marinade. Grill under a medium-high heat for 10 minutes, turning twice and each time brushing with marinade.

- Be careful not to overcook this dish – the delicious marinade will have made the lamb very tender and when served it should still be slightly pink right in the centre.

Mediterranean-Style Pork Casserole

(Serves 4; 8g fat and 275 calories per portion.)

Both pork and lamb cooked with fruit are delicious and this recipe is typical of many found in the eastern Mediterranean and north Africa.

450g (1lb) lean pork fillet, cubed
1 medium onion, chopped
16 dried apricots, 'no need to soak' variety
8 stoned prunes, 'no need to soak' variety
(or you can use dried apple rings)
2 whole cloves
1/2 cinnamon stick or 1 teaspoon ground cinnamon
Salt and black pepper
1 small glass dry white wine
A little chicken stock
1 level tablespoon plain flour

Arrange the pork cubes and onion in a casserole dish and add the fruit, spices and seasoning. Pour over the wine and then add stock to barely cover. Sieve the flour over the casserole. Cook at 150°C (300°F, gas mark 2) for 1 hour, stirring halfway through cooking time.

Before serving, remove the whole spices and check the seasoning.

- If the casserole is too dry, add a little more warm chicken stock and stir in before serving.
- You can make this dish using lean fillet of lamb, in which case it is 9 g fat and 295 calories per portion.

Mexican Chicken Fajitas

(Serves 4; 15g fat and 400 calories per portion.)

Mexican food is impressive but quite quick to put together.

2 chicken breast fillets, skinned and cut into strips
Juice of 1 lime
1 green chilli, de-seeded and finely chopped
1 tablespoon corn oil
1 medium red onion, sliced
1 large red pepper, de-seeded and chopped
1 large green pepper, de-seeded and chopped
1 clove garlic, chopped
Chopped parsley or coriander
8 wheat tortillas (Mexican pancakes), ready made
100ml (3½ fl oz) low-fat crème fraîche
1 (4–8 serving) quantity Salsa (see recipe page 101)

Put the chicken strips in a bowl and add the lime juice and the chilli. Stir well and leave for an hour or so.

Heat the oil in a non-stick pan and stir-fry the onion and pepper until soft and golden. Add the garlic, parsley and chicken plus marinade and stir-fry for a few minutes. Meanwhile, heat the tortillas.

When the chicken is cooked, top each portion with the crème fraîche and serve with the pancakes and salsa.

Moussaka

(Serves 4; 20.5g fat and 410 calories per portion.)

Moussaka is enjoying a bit of a revival in popularity. The traditional version soaks up masses of oil but this is much less grease-laden and, I think, nicer.

2 medium aubergines
2 tablespoons olive oil
2 medium onions, finely chopped
1 clove garlic, chopped
400g (14oz) lean lamb braising steak, minced
Pinch cinnamon
1 teaspoon dried oregano
Salt and black pepper
1 level tablespoon tomato purée
150ml (1/4 pint) beef stock
1 size 3 egg
1 (4-serving) quantity Cheese Sauce
(see recipe page 99)
2 tablespoons breadcrumbs
2 tablespoons Parmesan cheese

Slice the aubergines into rounds, brush with 1 tablespoon of the oil and grill or dry-fry for 5 minutes each side until golden; set aside.

Heat the remaining oil in a non-stick frying pan and stir-fry the onion until soft. Add garlic and lamb and stir until browned. Add the seasoning, tomato purée and stock and simmer for 30 minutes. Transfer the lamb mixture into baking dish; smooth the top. Cover with the aubergine slices and then beat the egg into the cheese sauce and spoon over the aubergines. Finally, mix the breadcrumbs with the Parmesan and sprinkle over the cheese sauce.

Bake at 190°C (375°F, gas mark 5) for 45 minutes.

- The moussaka is rich so it needs only a green salad and some boiled potatoes to accompany it.
- It is best to buy the leanest lamb braising steak and either mince it yourself or get the butcher to do it for you. Ready-minced lamb which you can buy in most supermarkets is higher in fat.

Piquant Pan-Fried Fish

(Serves 4; 9.5g fat and 270 calories per portion.)

Use any fish fillet or steak for this dish – but my favourites are swordfish and fresh tuna.

4 × 275g (10oz) fish portions
2 tablespoons olive oil
Juice of 2 lemons
4 tablespoons chopped parsley
(preferably flat-leaved parsley)
1 small onion, very finely chopped
1 clove garlic, chopped (optional)
Salt and black pepper

Place the fish in a large flat dish. Mix rest of ingredients together and tip over the fish, lifting the fish and spreading the marinade evenly around. Cover and leave in the fridge to marinate for an hour.

When ready to cook, transfer the fish and all the marinade into frying pan/s and fry over a medium heat for about 5 minutes each side (more if thick fish steaks are used).

Pizza Potatoes

(Serves 4; 13.5g fat and 425 calories per portion.)

A quick supper dish that children and adults alike enjoy.

4 × 225g (8oz) old, waxy potatoes, scrubbed and cut lengthways into 8 wedges each
8 extra lean bacon rashers, each cut into 2
1 (4-serving) quantity Tomato Sauce (see recipe page 102)
100g (3½oz) grated mozzarella
1 tablespoon chopped fresh parsley

Boil the potato pieces until barely cooked – about 8 minutes – and carefully drain and transfer to a large shallow baking dish. Meanwhile, grill or dry-fry the bacon and, when crisp, arrange in between the potato pieces. Pour over the tomato sauce, sprinkle on the cheese and grill under a medium heat for 5 minutes or until the cheese is bubbling.

Serve garnished with parsley.

- If you're in a real hurry and have no tomato sauce ready prepared, you can use a ready-made jar of Italian pasta sauce or pizza topping.
- Use ham or 2 × 185g cans tuna in brine (drained) for a change, instead of the bacon. Or you could use 200g (7oz) corned beef cut into chunks for the same calorie and fat count.

Prawn and Mushroom Risotto

(Serves 4; 7.5g fat and 405 calories per portion.)

1 tablespoon olive oil
1 medium onion or 8 shallots, finely chopped
275g (10oz) (dry weight) risotto rice
1 clove garlic, chopped
325g (12oz) mixed mushrooms – e.g. chestnut and shii-take – sliced
1.1 litres (2 pints) chicken stock, hot
225g (8oz) peeled prawns
1 large fresh tomato, chopped
1 small green pepper, de-seeded and chopped
1 teaspoon dried oregano
50ml (2 fl oz) dry white wine
Salt and black pepper
2 tablespoons Parmesan cheese

Heat the oil in a large non-stick frying pan and stir fry the onion or shallots until golden. Add the rice and garlic and stir. Add the mushrooms and stir for a minute with a little of the stock. Add the rest of the ingredients except the Parmesan, but reserving a little of the stock. Simmer very slowly, covered, until all the stock is absorbed. Test a spoonful of the rice – if it is still not cooked, add rest of stock and simmer again. The final risotto should not be too dry and the rice should be very soft but still in separate grains. This usually takes around 45 minutes.

Serve with the Parmesan cheese.

- The stock quantity given is only approximate as the water content of the ingredients – especially the mushrooms – varies a lot.

- You can use chopped turkey instead of the prawns. If the turkey is raw, add it to the pan with the onion.

Savoury Pancakes

(Serves 4; 5g fat and 225 calories per portion.)

This quantity makes eight pancakes – which can be frozen layered in between greaseproof paper.

175g (6oz) plain flour
100ml (3½ fl oz) water
175ml (6 fl oz) skimmed milk
2 size 4 eggs
Salt and black pepper
25g (1oz) low-fat spread

Mix all the ingredients except the low-fat spread in a bowl and beat well. Heat a small non-stick frying pan with a little of the low-fat spread and brush over the base to coat. When the pan is nice and hot, add one-eighth of the pancake mixture and quickly tip the pan so that it covers the base completely in a thin layer. After a minute, slide a heatproof spatula under the pancake and check if it is golden. If it is, toss or turn and cook other side for 30 seconds.

Turn out on to a plate and keep warm while you make seven more pancakes, each time brushing the pan with a little more spread. Use as required (e.g. recipe page 132).

- If you have a really good, heavyweight small non-stick frying pan you could save even more fat by using Fry Light spray instead of the low-fat spread.

Salmon and Broccoli Pancakes

(Serves 4; 21g fat and 525 calories per portion.)

8 Savoury Pancakes (see recipe page 131)
1 (4-serving) quantity Cheese Sauce (see recipe page 99)
300g (11oz) salmon fillet, skin removed
225g (8oz) broccoli head, cut into very small florets
50ml (2 fl oz) skimmed milk
2 tablespoons Parmesan cheese
Finely chopped parsley

Keep the pancakes and cheese sauce warm.

Microwave or poach the salmon fillet in water until just cooked – this will only take a few minutes. Flake it gently. Steam, microwave or boil the broccoli florets until barely tender, drain and cool. Mix half the cheese sauce with the salmon and broccoli. Put 4 tablespoons of the mixture in the centre of each pancake and roll up, laying the filled pancakes side by side in an oblong baking dish. Beat the skimmed milk into the remaining cheese sauce with half the Parmesan and pour over the pancakes.

Sprinkle the remaining Parmesan over and place under medium grill for five minutes until the top is golden and bubbling.

Serve garnished with parsley.

- You can use ready-made cannelloni rings instead of the pancakes in this recipe if you like, following the instructions on the packet for cooking the cannelloni.
- The salmon and broccoli mixture is also nice in a seafood lasagne.

- Pancakes and cannelloni can also be filled with the Bolognese mixture (see recipe page 97) or the chilli mixture (see recipe page 121) and topped with Tomato Sauce (see recipe page 102) or a cheese sauce as in this recipe.

Salmon Brochettes with Wild Rice

(Serves 4; 20.5g fat and 465 calories per portion.)

Salmon is a fairly high-fat dish – but its fat content is primarily the 'good for you' kind – and salmon tastes so rich that a little goes a long way.

4 × 125g (4½oz) salmon fillets, each cut into 10 cubes
1 tablespoon olive oil
2 tablespoons Lea and Perrins Ginger and Orange sauce
Salt and black pepper
4 small courgettes, cut into 1 inch (2.5 cm) slices
16 button mushrooms
225g (8oz) easy cook long grain and wild rice

Soak 8 small wooden skewers in water overnight (or use metal ones). Place salmon chunks in a bowl with the oil, ginger and orange, with seasoning and leave for an hour or so to marinade.

Thread salmon, courgettes and mushrooms on to the skewers and brush with marinade. Put the rice on to boil in a lidded saucepan as instructed on packet.

Heat the grill and grill the brochettes for around 10 minutes until a medium-high heat until cooked, turning once or twice during cooking and basting with leftover marinade.

Serve with the rice.

- The brochettes go well with a leafy green salad including some rocket and frisee lettuce.
- If you like you can serve everyone with a half portion of Salsa (see recipe page 101) with this dish, adding 1.75g fat and 24 calories per serving.
- You can also make the brochettes with monkfish to reduce the fat content further.

Spanish Tortilla

(Serves 4; 13g fat and 215 calories per portion.)

This is a fairly authentic version of a Spanish omelette which will soon oust egg and chips as the family's favourite supper.

1 tablespoon corn oil
225g (8oz) potato, parboiled
1 medium onion, thinly sliced
1 clove garlic, chopped (optional)
1 red pepper, de-seeded and thinly sliced
6 size 3 eggs
1 tablespoon chopped fresh parsley
Salt and black pepper

Heat the oil in a large non-stick frying pan and slice the potato into rounds. Add them to the pan and fry a few minutes either side until golden. Remove with a slotted spatula. Add the onion, garlic (if used) and pepper to the pan and stir-fry for a few minutes until golden and soft. Return the potatoes to the pan, distributing them evenly over the onion and peppers.

Beat the eggs in a bowl with the parsley and seasoning and pour over the vegetables in the pan. Cook over a medium heat for 5 minutes, then either invert the omelette carefully using two spatulas and cook other side for 2 minutes *or* (and I prefer this way) place the omelette in the pan under a medium grill and cook for 3–4 minutes until the top is golden.

Cut into wedges and serve.

- This is also nice served cold in place of a high-fat quiche.
- You can use thinly sliced courgettes instead of the peppers in this dish (or half and half) for a change.

Turkey and Noodle Stir-Fry

(Serves 4; 7.25g fat and 440 calories per portion.)

Egg noodles make a delicious change from rice and are much quicker to cook.

275g (10oz) (dry weight) medium egg noodles
1 tablespoon groundnut or corn oil
350g (12oz) lean stir-fry turkey
225g (8oz) broccoli, cut into small florets
1 yellow pepper, de-seeded and cut into strips
100g (3½oz) mushrooms, sliced
8 spring onions, cut in half
1 small piece ginger
110ml (4 fl oz) chicken stock
1 tablespoon dry sherry
1 tablespoon soya sauce
2 teaspoons cornflour
Salt if necessary

Bring a large pan of water to the boil and add the noodles. Remove the pan from heat and leave noodles to soak for 6 minutes. Drain and reserve.

Heat the oil in a large non-stick frying pan and stir-fry the turkey and broccoli for a few minutes until the turkey is tinged gold. Add the pepper, mushrooms, onion and ginger and stir-fry for a further 3 minutes, adding a little chicken stock if necessary. Add the sherry and bubble. Add the soya sauce. Mix the cornflour with the remaining stock and add to pan; bubble for one minute.

Add the noodles to the pan, mix gently and serve.

- You can use lean beef or chicken instead of turkey; add 2g fat and 30 calories for the beef, and 1g fat and 15 calories for the chicken, per portion.

Roast Selection of Vegetables

(Serves 4; approximately 3.75g fat and 90 calories per portion, depending on vegetables chosen.)

Ideal for people who aren't so keen on plain boiled vegetables – this cooking method will convert anyone!

Choose a selection of around four of the following vegetables to a total weight of 650g–1kg ($1^1/_2$–$1^3/_4$lb):

- *Aubergine*
- *Carrot*
- *Courgettes*
- *Fennel bulbs*
- *Onion*
- *Parsnip*
- *Peppers – red, yellow or orange*
- *Swede*
- *Sweet potato*
- *Turnip*

Then you will need:

- *1 tablespoon olive or corn oil*
- *Salt and black pepper*
- *Some fresh rosemary and thyme sprigs (optional)*
- *A few cloves of garlic (optional)*

All you have to do is cut the vegetables into quarters (fennel, peppers), eighths (onion) or batons (most root vegetables and aubergines), whichever is most appropriate. Toss them in a bowl with the oil and seasoning then lay out flat on a roasting tin. Place the herb sprigs and garlic (unpeeled) amongst them and roast for about 40 minutes or until coloured and tender.

- A good winter selection is root vegetables plus Spanish or English onion. A good summer selection is peppers, aubergine and courgettes plus red onion.
- Cut carrots slightly smaller than the other roots as they take longer to roast.
- Halved tomatoes can be added to the summer selection if you like.
- Garlic cloves roasted in their skins have a mild nutty flavour – not at all like raw garlic.

Tomato Rice

(Serves 4; trace of fat and 280 calories per portion.)

If you're having a plain grill, a saucy savoury rice makes a more interesting accompaniment than plain boiled rice.

275g (10oz) (dry weight) long grain rice, e.g. Basmati
1 × 400g can chopped tomatoes
1 small onion, finely chopped
450ml ($^3/_4$ pint) vegetable stock
1 small carrot, grated
Juice of 1 orange
1 level teaspoon ground cumin
Salt and black pepper

Place all ingredients in a saucepan and simmer, covered, for 20 minutes or until liquid is absorbed and rice is tender.

- The finished rice dish shouldn't be *too* dry, so if towards the end of the cooking time it does look dry, add a little boiling water to the pan.

PUDDINGS

Chocolate Pear Delight

(Serves 4; 6g fat and 95 calories per portion.)

Chocolate and pears are a marvellous combination – and this dessert tastes much more 'wicked' than it really is!

4 cooking pears, e.g. Conference
1 tablespoon fruit sugar
2 teaspoons water
8 tablespoon aerosol chocolate mousse
8 tablespoons aerosol cream
1 level teaspoon cocoa powder

Peal and slice the pears lengthways into eighths. If you have a microwave, place the pears in an oval dish with the sugar and water, cover and cook on high for 3–4 minutes or until tender. Otherwise, poach the pears in a small saucepan with the sugar and water.

Divide the pears and their liquid between four glass serving dishes – small sundae glasses are ideal – then swirl on first the chocolate, then the cream aerosol. Top with the cocoa powder.

- If you can't get aerosol chocolate mousse, instead use 1 scoop of WeightWatchers chocolate ice cream on each dish – the calorie count will be very slightly higher.

Filo Fruit Pie

(Serves 4; 7.25g fat and 190 calories per portion.)

I actually now prefer the light crunchy taste and texture of filo in baking to traditional shortcrust pastry – and it is so much easier than making your own pastry – just brush and bake!

450–500g (1lb–1lb 2oz) mixed fruits of choice – e.g. apple and blackberry
2 level tablespoons fruit sugar
6 sheets Jus Rol filo pastry
25g (1oz) butter
1 teaspoon fruit sugar to finish

Wash, peel and chop the fruits as necessary and place in saucepan or microwave and soften (but don't cook thoroughly), stirring once or twice. Add two level teaspoons of fruit sugar. Soft fruits take a few minutes, pears, apples, etc. a few minutes more.

Put the sweetened fruit and any juices in a square baking dish and leave to cool slightly. Make sure the pastry is thawed and covered. Melt the butter carefully and, taking one sheet of filo at a time from the cover, brush very lightly with the butter and arrange on top of the fruit, scrunching each sheet slightly. Make sure the pastry covers the top of the pie completely by the time you've laid on all six sheets, and press down the edges on to the dish. Use up any remaining butter by brushing on to the top layer, and bake at 200°C (400°F, gas mark 6) for 20 minutes or until top is golden and crisp.

Sprinkle the remaining sugar on top.

- You can use all soft fruits in this pie – or try pears and raspberries, or peaches and apricots. The sweeter the fruit is naturally, the less fruit sugar you will need to use – it is easy to test for sweetness after softening and before you put the fruit in the pie dish.

Pineapple Brûleé

(Serves 4; 1.5g fat and 120 calories per portion.)

You will need four small ramekins for this dish.

100ml (3½ fl oz) low-fat Greek yogurt
150ml (¼ pint) low-fat custard
Grated rind of 1 lemon
1 × 400g can pineapple pieces or chunks, drained
2 tablespoons fruit sugar

Mix together the yogurt, custard and lemon rind. Divide the pineapple pieces between the ramekins and cover each with a quarter of the custard mixture. Sprinkle the sugar evenly over the top of all four and grill under a medium heat until golden and bubbling.

Serve hot or cold.

Raspberry Layer

(Serves 4; 5.6g fat and 130 calories per portion.)

325g (12oz) fresh or frozen raspberries
2 tablespoons fruit sugar
450ml (¾ pint) low-fat Greek strained yogurt

In a medium saucepan over a low heat, heat the raspberries until they have made some pourable juice – about two or three tablespoons. Drain off the excess juice and reserve. Mix half the fruit sugar in with this reserved juice and the other half in the raspberries, stirring very gently for a second or two only (to keep the raspberries from breaking up).

Using four small sundae dishes, put a tablespoon of the yogurt into each dish then top each with a quarter of the raspberries. Divide the rest of the yogurt between the four dishes. Finish by pouring the reserved juice over the dishes.

Chill and serve.

OPTIONS AND FILLINGS

Baked Potato Fillings and Toast Toppings

Group 1

- Scoop out half the cooked potato and leave to cool slightly; mix in 25g (1oz) Promise low-fat spread and return to potato. Top with 25g (1oz) grated or sliced mozzarella cheese and sliced tomato and grill for 30 seconds.
- 50g (2oz) low-fat soft cheese mixed with 25g (1oz) lean ham, chopped and 2 spring onions, chopped – warm under grill.
- 1 portion Salsa (see recipe page 101) plus 15g ($^1/_2$oz) low-fat Cheddar cheese, grated.
- 1 size 3 egg and 50g (2oz) canned red pepper, chopped, scrambled with seasoning and 1 tablespoon skimmed milk in a non-stick saucepan.

- 25g (1oz) low-fat crème fraîche mixed with 1 level teaspoon Dijon mustard or a little curry powder and 1 slice lean back bacon, grilled and crumbled.
- 1 size 3 egg and 50g (2oz) button mushrooms, sliced, all poached in a little seasoned water, plus 15g low-fat spread.

Group 2

- Half portion Chilli Beef Pizza topping (see recipe page 94).
- Half portion Bolognese sauce (see recipe page 97).
- One-third portion Chilli Con Carne (see recipe page 121).

Group 3

- 75g (3oz) smoked haddock fillet, poached, drained and flaked and mixed with 2 tablespoons Cheese Sauce (see recipe page 99). Top potato or toast, heat and serve.
- 50g (2oz) tuna in brine, drained and mixed with 1 chopped tomato and 25g (1oz) drained cannellini beans plus 1 tablespoon Kraft Free Choice 1,000 Island-style dressing or oil-free French dressing.
- 100g (3½oz) soft cod's roes, microwaved on medium until just cooked or poached in 1 tablespoon water.

Group 4

- 100g (3½oz) baked beans, barbecue *or* chilli *or* with bacon.
- 150g (5½oz) baked beans in tomato sauce.
- 150 g (5½ oz) spaghetti in tomato sauce.
- 1 portion Roast Vegetables (see recipe page 136) topped with 15g (½oz) grated half-fat Cheddar cheese.

- 1 portion Tomato Sauce (see recipe page 102) with 15g ($^{1}/_{2}$oz) low-fat Cheddar cheese, grated.

Bread Fillings

Group 1

- 40g ($1^{1}/_{2}$oz) Tartare Light cheese and 25g (1oz) lean ham.
- 15g ($^{1}/_{2}$oz) Tartare Light mixed with 15g ($^{1}/_{2}$oz) full-fat Cheddar cheese, grated and 25g (1oz) pineapple pieces.
- 40g ($1^{1}/_{2}$oz) half-fat Cheddar cheese *or* Brie *or* Edam plus tomato.
- 1 size 3 egg, hard boiled and sliced, plus 2 teaspoons Kraft Free Choice mayonnaise-style dressing and cress or cucumber.

Group 2

- 1 × 50g (2oz) lean beefburger, grilled plus 1 teaspoon relish or salsa.
- 2 average (vacuum-packed type) slices chicken *or* turkey *or* smoked turkey *or* lean ham *or* pork *or* roast beef plus 1 tablespoon stuffing *or* relish *or* reduced-calorie mayonnaise.
- 1 average slice corned beef plus 2 teaspoons sweet pickle.
- 2 vacuum-packed slices tongue and sliced tomato.
- 25g (1oz) liver sausage with 2 teaspoons pickle or fruit sauce.
- 3 vacuum-packed slices lean ham plus mustard.
- BLT: 2 × 25g (1oz) (average thin slices from vacuum pack) extra lean bacon, grilled until crisp, plus sliced iceberg lettuce, sliced tomato and 2 teaspoons Kraft Free Choice mayonnaise-style dressing.

- 2 low-fat pork and beef chipolatas, well grilled and sliced plus 2 teaspoons fruity or other bottled relish or mustard.

Group 3

- Prawn cocktail – 60g (2$^{1}/_{2}$oz) peeled prawns *or* mixed ready-prepared frozen seafood, defrosted, plus 2 teaspoons reduced-calorie mayonnaise and thinly sliced iceberg lettuce.
- 2 sardines canned in brine, drained, plus 2 teaspoons Kraft Free Choice mayonnaise-style dressing *or* 2 teaspoons tomato sauce.
- 75g (3 oz) tuna in brine *or* 50g (2oz) pink salmon, drained, plus 2 teaspoons Free Choice mayonnaise *or* 1,000 Island-style dressing.
- 1 × 43g can dressed crabmeat, drained, plus 2 teaspoons Kraft Free Choice mayonnaise-style dressing.
- 1 portion Smoked Trout Pâté (see recipe page 93) plus sliced tomato and cucumber.

Group 4

- Marmite and cucumber.
- 1 medium banana, mashed with 1 teaspoon runny honey and a dash of lemon juice.
- 25g (1oz) Tartex Vegetable Pâté.
- 1 × 50g (2oz) Vegeburger made from dry mix without added egg plus 1 teaspoon relish of choice.
- 2 level tablespoons hummus.

Don't forget that chopped, fresh salad items can be added to any of these fillings and toppings as you like – the more the better.

CHAPTER 6

Take Thirty!

A simple action plan to get that body fat moving!

> *Note:* This plan is for people in normal health. If you have any physical disability or illness that you think may prevent you from exercising, then show your doctor this programme before beginning and get his or her approval.

Take just thirty minutes a day, five days a week – and, even if you're unfit and haven't taken any exercise in years, you could easily be walking ten miles or more a week *within* weeks!

You've attacked the fat in your food – and by doing so, you're already shedding body fat steadily – so now let's attack your body fat directly – by burning it off with some regular activity of the right kind.

Most people are put off taking more exercise – even though they know they should – either because they fear they are too unfit even to start, or because they think it will be complicated, time-consuming or boring.

The plan I've devised is simple, easy for anyone in normal health to do and *the* most effective way to burn off your body fat within reasonable time limits.

It's based on walking. But first let's look at some of the terrific bonuses that doing some regular exercise (of the right kind) can achieve:

- It's good for your figure. Each time you do a *Take Thirty* exercise session you'll be burning some extra body fat – enough to help you shed up to a *stone* (6.5 kg) of surplus fat a year, over and above what you're shedding through a reduced-fat diet. If you *don't* need to shed that much weight, don't worry; you needn't get over-thin. You can just eat a little more to compensate.
- It keeps your bones strong. Regular weight-bearing exercise such as walking helps keep your bones dense and can help prevent osteoporosis and fractures in later life.
- It helps keep your heart healthy. A lifestyle that is too sedentary is a well-known risk factor for heart disease and strokes. Physical activity is protective in several ways – it helps lower the concentration of 'LDL' cholesterol (the kind that is clearly linked with heart disease) in the blood. It reduces blood pressure. And in improving stamina, it makes your heart stronger and able to work with less effort.
- It helps you feel better. Because the right kind of activity oxygenates your body – literally carrying life-giving oxygen to every pore – you have an enhanced sense of well-being. You feel more alert, more lively, and yet more relaxed after regular sessions. Remember I mentioned in chapter 1 that one of the risk factors

for heart disease can be high levels of stress – well, here is a simple way to dissipate stress while attacking the fat!

These are just some of the reasons why the *Take Thirty* plan can help your health and your body and why I want you to try it. Here is all I want you to do.

I want you to find thirty minutes of your time and put it aside for yourself and your body five *times a week and I want you to use that time to walk.*

That's all. In a minute I'll be explaining the few, easy instructions you need to know, but first let's look at that time I want you to find.

Finding thirty

If you've spent years leading a very busy life and not bothering to take much exercise – or, even, like one in six of our UK population, none at all – you may at first think that to find 30 minutes to exercise is asking too much.

If that sounds like you then we have to look at your priorities. Here are some questions to ask yourself.

- Is 2½ hours a week spent on helping my body to health less important than the two or three TV programmes I watched but didn't really enjoy? (Or think of something else you did this week that you didn't really enjoy – say you read a paperback you found quite boring.)
- If I can find time for the hairdressers, to go shopping, to chat on the phone, to have a lie-in, then why can't I find time to keep my body fit?

You can see what I'm getting at. Not only do we make time for the things we consider important, we frequently *waste* time of things that aren't important at all.

If you accept that taking more physical exercise *is* important for you and your well-being – then you can find time.

Because the activity I am asking you to do – walking – is so easy and can be done anywhere, you can also probably make 'extra' time for it much more easily than for any other activity. For instance, if you think of your 30 minutes as 15 minutes *out* and 15 minutes *back* you could use it to do any of the following:

- Take a packed lunch to work, walk 15 minutes to the park (or any suitable outdoor eating site), eat, then walk 15 minutes back.
- Walk your child to school if it is approximately a 15-minute journey.
- Walk to the shops if you only need a few items rather than taking the car.
- Instead of driving or taking the bus to the station if you commute, walk to the station and back again in the evening. (Splitting your walk into two separate sessions like that isn't ideal but it is certainly better than not doing the walk.)

Right. The thing to do now is decide when you are going to fit the five *Take Thirty* sessions in to your week – and then, barring illness, emergencies, accidents, or genuine reasons not to do it, *stick* to those times.

Believe me, from experience – *if you don't forward plan, you probably won't do it.*

Here are some guidelines to bear in mind when doing this forward planning:

- Space your five *Take Thirty* sessions out evenly during the week. Don't, for instance, do three in one day and nothing for the next five days!

- Decide not only when but where you're going to walk. Flat walking is ideal to start with, especially if you are unfit. If you do have time and access to a vehicle you could always vary your route by driving to a new starting point.
- Winter walking. Try not to walk alone after dark in isolated (or dangerously busy traffic) areas. Do your best to fit your walk into daylight hours. If this really is not possible, walk on your days off and find an alternative (see page 158) for the other days until spring arrives.

Now some practicalities.

What to wear

- Wear suitable-weight clothes for the time of year, bearing in mind that if you are walking to burn fat you will get hot during your walk. 'Layers' are best. You can always take a small light rucksack in which to put discarded clothes – and even a drink.
- Wear clothes that don't restrict your movement – a tight skirt is not the answer! A tracksuit is ideal for colder months and shirt and shorts for the summer. Keep your neck and shoulders covered in sunny warm weather. A brimmed hat is a good idea.
- Wear comfortable shoes that offer cushioned support – for most people the best bet is trainers. Socks are important will protect your feet even more.

How to walk

This isn't as ridiculous as it sounds – we all know how to walk, don't we? But for fat-burning and for maximum health benefits, you need to follow these simple guidelines:

- Take the first three minutes to warm up. Start off at a moderate pace, breathing normally and swinging your arms gently. By the end of three minutes you should feel warm.
- For the majority of your walk, concentrate on travelling at as brisk a pace as you can comfortably go *without* getting so breathless that you have to stop, or couldn't talk. Your stride will naturally lengthen to accommodate this increased pace and your arms will be swinging quite strongly.

If at any time you find yourself 'puffing and panting' you should slow back down until your breathing is as above – and if at any time you realize that you aren't breathing more deeply than usual you should increase the pace until you do. What you are aiming for is controlled exertion that is slightly or moderately hard but not difficult. You will be aware of your heart beating and your lungs working harder than usual but you don't feel discomfort.

This is the pace at which you will begin burning fat, and towards the end of your walk you will be burning more.

Remember – if you walk too slowly so that you're under-exerting, or too fast, so that you get breathless and have to stop, you *won't* be burning fat.

If you are not sure that you are going at the right pace, there is an easy pulse test you can do. All you need is a watch with a second hand. Simply stop (keep marching on the spot if possible to keep your heart rate constant) and immediately find your pulse in the angle between your jaw and your neck, using your first two fingers. Time 15 seconds and count the pulse beats during that 15 seconds. If the number of beats comes within the two sets of figures listed opposite your nearest age on the chart below, then you are walking at the correct pace for you to burn fat. If your count is lower than the lowest given for your age (the beginners' level), you are below your 'training zone' level and you should try a little harder; if your count is higher than the highest given for your age (the intermediate level), then you should slow down a little and test again in a few minutes. If you haven't exercised lately and would classify yourself as 'unfit', aim for the 'beginners' pulse rate for a few weeks and gradually improve to the 'intermediate' level.

- Take the last two minutes to cool down. As you finish your walk, slow the pace down to warm-up pace. When

PULSE RATE CHART

	Pulse count for 15 seconds	
AGE	BEGINNERS	INTERMEDIATE
20	30	35
25	29	34
30	28	33
35	28	32
40	27	31
45	26	30
50	25	30
55	25	29
60	24	28
65+	23	27

you have finished your walk you should ideally take a minute or two to stretch out your main leg muscles – this helps to prevent any muscular stiffness tomorrow.

Leg stretches

1. *Hamstring stretch*

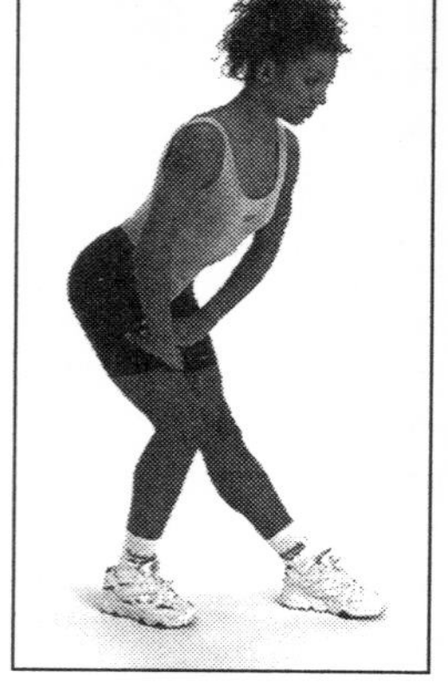

Stand with right foot approximately 12 inches (30 cm) behind left foot, right knee bent. Stretch left leg out straight, keeping foot flat on floor and bend over it, resting both hands on right thigh for support. Feeling a good stretch along the back of the thigh in the left leg, hold for a count of sixteen. Repeat position on the other side.

2. *Quad stretch*

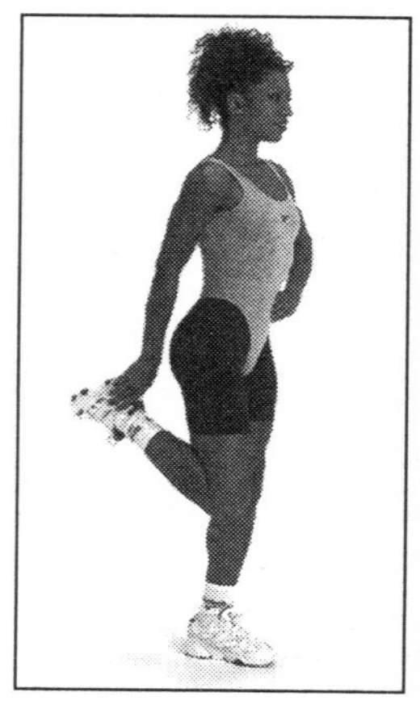

Stand with feet hip width apart, knees loose, tummy tucked in. Bring your right foot back, bending at knee, and clasp foot with right hand as shown. Feeling the stretch down the front of your right thigh, hold for a count of sixteen. Repeat position on the other side. Take care not to arch your back while doing this exercise.

3. Calf stretch

Stand with right foot approximately 12–18 inches (30–45 cm) behind left foot. Keep left foot flat and toes pointing forwards and body weight slightly forward of centre, right leg straight. Press right heel into floor and feel a stretch in the mid and upper calf. Hold for a count of sixteen. Repeat position on other side.

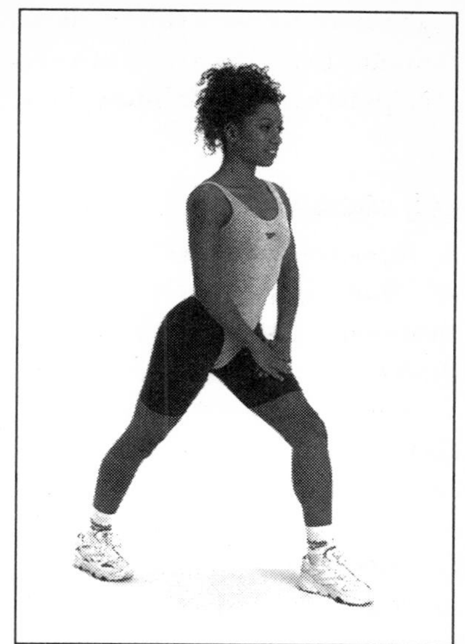

4. Lower calf stretch

Stand with right foot a few inches behind left foot, both knees bent and body weight over right leg. Bend right knee until you feel a stretch in the lower calf, keeping right heel on floor throughout. Hold for a count of sixteen. Repeat position on other side.

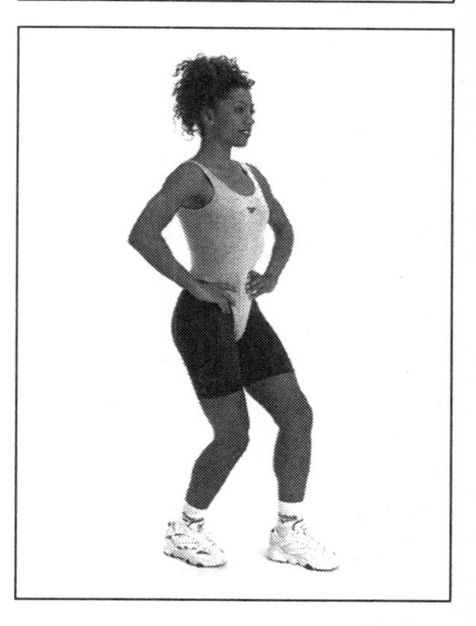

5. Shin stretch
Stand with one foot behind you, heel off floor and tops of toes resting on floor. Push toes down gently into the floor so that you feel a stretch all along top of foot and shin. Hold for a count of sixteen. Relax and repeat position with other foot.

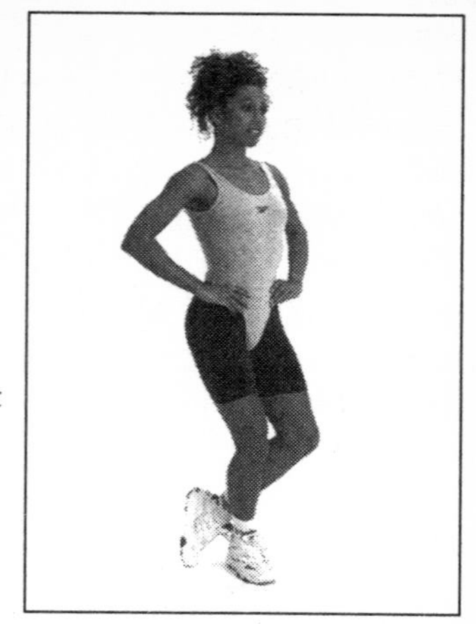

6. Ankle stretch
Stand and, placing the outside of your left foot on the floor behind your right leg and with left knee bent, curtsey, bending right knee slightly as you go. Hold the curtsey so that you feel a stretch along the outer side of your left ankle, for a count of sixteen. Relax and repeat position on the other side.

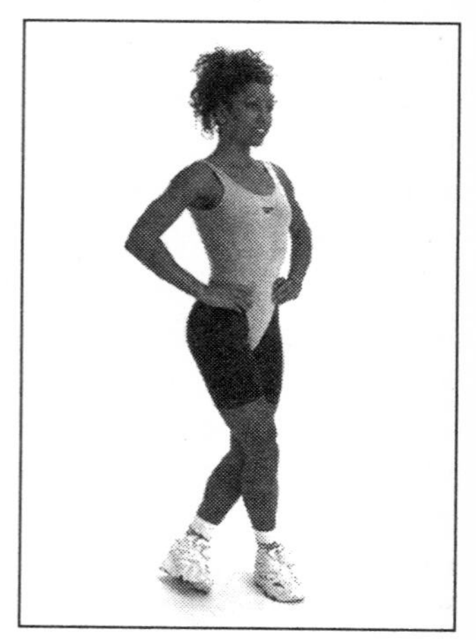

How it works

When you walk your lower body muscles are being asked to do extra work, for which they need energy. If you walk too slowly, so that your heart rate isn't increased, or too quickly, so that you become over-exerted, the fuel your muscles prefer to use is glycogen – a carbohydrate source of fuel. But with moderate-intensity work your muscles will begin to call upon your body's fat stores and use the fat for energy. The longer you keep up the moderate-intensity work, the higher the proportion of fat to glycogen burned. And the stronger your muscles become over weeks and months and years of regular walking, the better they get at burning that fat for fuel.

That's how walking helps you burn fat.

To get progressively fitter, though, you need to improve your walking.

Progressing

After you have been walking regularly for a week or two, you will notice that the pace at which you felt real effort for the first few sessions you now find easy. To achieve the same level of exertion, you now need to walk faster. This of course means that you will walk further in the allotted 30 minutes, and as the week go on and your heart and lungs get fitter and fitter, you will be able to walk further and further.

The chart overleaf gives a sample of the sort of progress that the average person (relatively unfit in week 1) can achieve. What is happening is that your lung capacity is improving so that you can take in more oxygen with each breath; and your heart muscle is stronger, so that it can pump more blood around your body with each beat.

Obviously if you keep improving there will come a time when you can't walk any faster without running. There is no need for the average person to get any fitter than this for the sake of his health or his size. However, for those who want to, two other ways to improve are to do more uphill walking, which is harder than working on the flat, or walk wearing light hand weights (not wrist weights). By adding weight to yourself, again you're giving your body more work to do.

However, for all practical purposes for most of us, by the time you've reached stage 6 on the chart – that is, the equivalent of walking at 5 mph for 30 minutes – you can then simply maintain that level to maintain your fitness.

Another alternative is simply to walk for longer periods – instead of 30 minutes, do 45-minutes or 1-hour walks – it's up to you! Remember – the *more* you walk (at the correct intensity) the *more* fat you will burn and the fitter you will get. The *Take Thirty* five times a week plan is plenty for most people but once you are fit there is nothing to stop you doing more.

THE TAKE THIRTY *WALKING CHART*

	Mon	Tue	Wed	Thur	Fri	Sat	Sun
Stage 1	1.0	—	1.0	1.0	—	1.0	1.0
Stage 2	1.5	—	1.5	1.5	—	1.5	1.5
Stage 3	1.75	—	1.75	1.75	—	1.75	1.75
Stage 4	2.0	—	2.0	2.0	—	2.0	2.0
Stage 5	2.25	—	2.25	2.25	—	2.25	2.25
Stage 6	2.5	—	2.5	2.5	—	2.5	2.5

(All figures are miles covered in 30 minutes.)

Most people in an average state of health should be able to move up to the next stage every week, so that after five weeks you have built up to 5 mph. However, this is nothing but a guide, and it could take you twice that time. Depending on your fitness level, your age and other factors you may, indeed, never reach stage 6 but find that stage 4 or 5 still gives you enough exertion.

You don't *need* to measure the distance you cover on this programme – only your own exertion. I've provided you with this chart for interest only. At no stage should you over-exert to try to cover a set distance in the allotted time. It's always best to maintain a pace that is within your own optimum pulse-rate limits.

Your first Take Thirty *walk*

Before we leave the *Take Thirty* walking programme I would like you to actually do your first walk. This is because some of you will find that you cannot manage to walk for 30 minutes at the moderate exertion pace I've described. Some of you may find your legs aching and/or that you are feeling tired when 10 or 15 minutes is up. That's OK. There is no need to feel ashamed or give up. Lots of people are in the same boat. You can improve your fitness level, believe me, so that within weeks you will be walking quicker and further than you ever thought you could.

All you have to do is go out on the prescribed days and walk for as long as you feel able. Soon – maybe next week, maybe in a month's time – you will be able to start on stage 1. If you are extremely unfit you could even start with three sessions a week and build up to the five. Do what feels right for you and remember the most important thing is striking a balance between what you can achieve without discomfort and accepting that in order to improve you *do* have to put some effort in.

ALTERNATIVES TO WALKING

There will be occasions when you can't walk – the weather is too bad or it is too dark, perhaps. All the following are an acceptable alternative:

- *Fat Attack* video fat-burning section (see last page of book for details)
- Swimming
- Exercise bike
- Treadmill
- Aerobics class
- Dancing (upbeat)
- Step workout

All the above should be done at a pace that gives you the correct pulse rate for you, of course, as explained earlier.

BODY-CONDITIONING

The *Take Thirty* walking programme will tone up your lower body muscles very well – you will, over the weeks and months, see an improvement in the shape of your bottom, thighs and calves, and to a lesser extent your hips. If you're walking with correct posture – tummy tucked in – your stomach should also flatten out.

You can add the following short routine to your walking programme, if you like, to give a complete all-over body-toning effect – do the exercises after your walk or at another suitable time of day. If you do the routine on returning from your walk, you need NOT do the warm-up exercises, but you should still do the warm-up stretches (except stretches 5 and 6) in addition to your leg stretches.

Wear comfortable non-restrictive clothes.

Warm-up

Unless instructed otherwise, stand with feet hip-width apart, tummy tucked in, shoulders and knees relaxed and toes pointing forward. Breathe normally throughout.

1. Remembering to keep your posture correct (as above), roll both shoulders backwards in a circular motion, keeping arms relaxed. Repeat eight times, then reverse to roll them forwards and repeat eight times.
2. Now make bigger circles with alternate arms, keeping arms loose and raising elbows a little higher than shoulder level. Circle alternate arms backwards eight times each, then forwards eight times each.
3. Now march on the stop, swinging arms as you go, sixteen times.
4. Right – now, knee lifts. Start with much of your weight over your right foot, then bring your left knee up and across your body, bringing your right elbow down towards your left knee as you go. In a flowing motion, repeat to other side and repeat sixteen times.
5. Now march on the spot again, arms swinging, sixteen times.
6. Keeping plenty of movement going, bring each heel behind you and up towards your bottom, feeling your hamstrings work. Do sixteen of these on alternate legs, keeping the rhythm going.

7. Okay – now take a step to the right and bring your left leg to meet the right leg. Step to the left and take your right leg to meet left leg. As you step to the right, bring left arm up and reach for the ceiling. As you step to the left, bring right arm up in the same way. Keep this up in a good rhythm for a count of sixteen.
8. Continue stepping to each side as in 7, but this time add the following arm movement: place arms to the side and, keeping upper arms parallel to the floor, squeeze forearms together and release on each step, to feel your chest working.

Repeat the whole sequence from 3–8.

Now let's go into some warm-up stretches. Hold each stretch for a count of eight.

1. Stand with one leg forward and one leg back. Take weight over front leg and feel the stretch in the calf of the back leg. At the same time, take opposite arm (to back leg) up and over head, bent at elbow so palm lies behind your neck. Using the other hand, press gently on elbow to stretch your tricep. Repeat stretch with other leg and tricep.

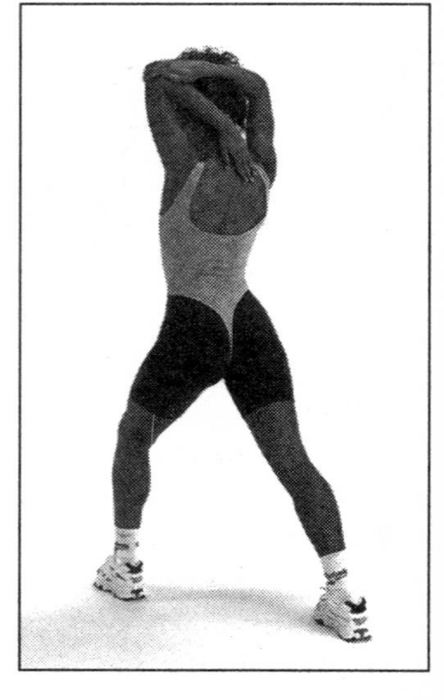

2. Take feet apart approximately 12–18 inches (30–45cm), keeping them parallel. Bend knees and lean forward, resting hands on thighs. Round your lower back, pulling tummy in to a count of four, then release to a count of four.

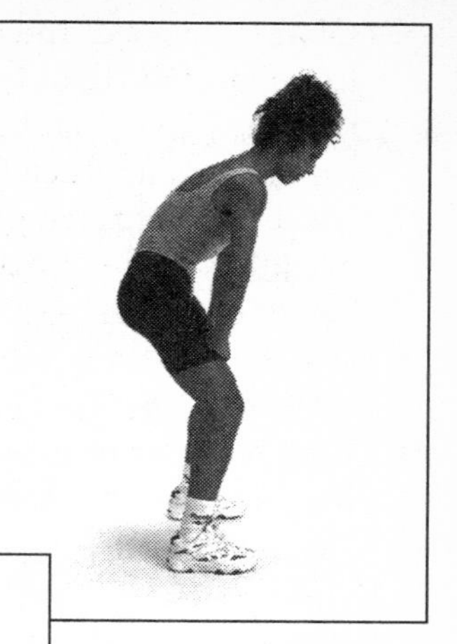

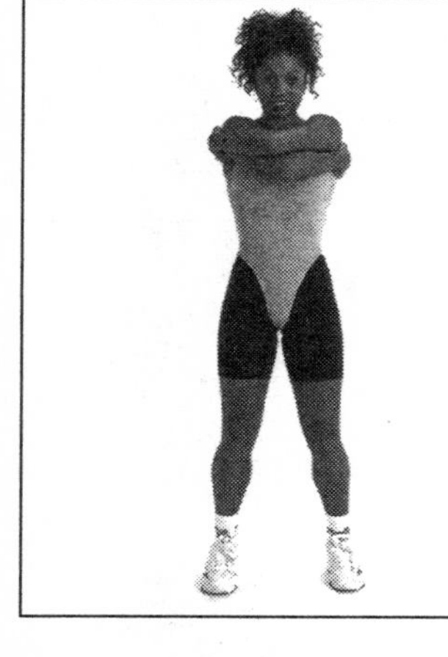

3. Return to upright position and cross arms over your chest. Give yourself a hug!

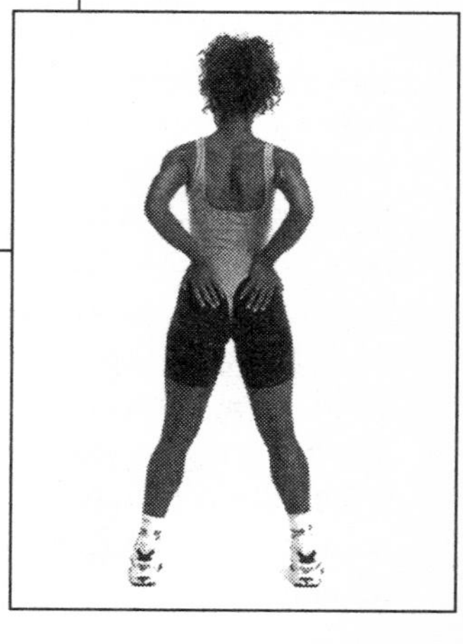

4. Place your hands flat on the back of your hips. Now squeeze elbows together, keeping shoulders down. Remember to count eight while you hold.

5. Now bring feet together and stand with tummy tucked in, knees loose. Now pick up right foot, bend at knee and take foot behind you as shown. Hold and repeat with left leg.

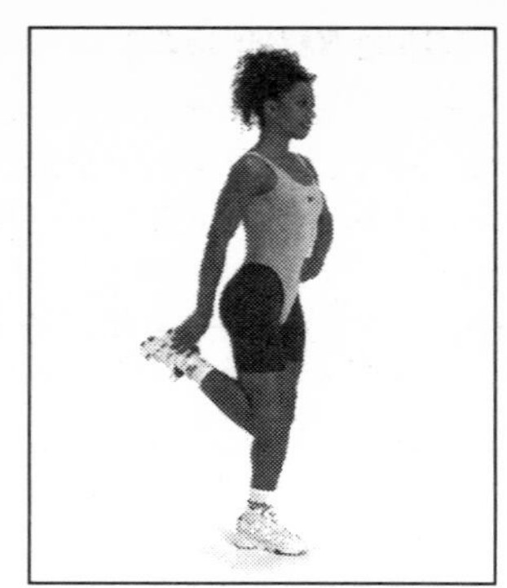

6. Now with left leg forward, right leg back and left knee bent, this time transfer weight over left leg and, keeping your body forward over the left leg and placing hands on left thigh, feel the stretch along the back of your right thigh (hamstring). Repeat to other side.

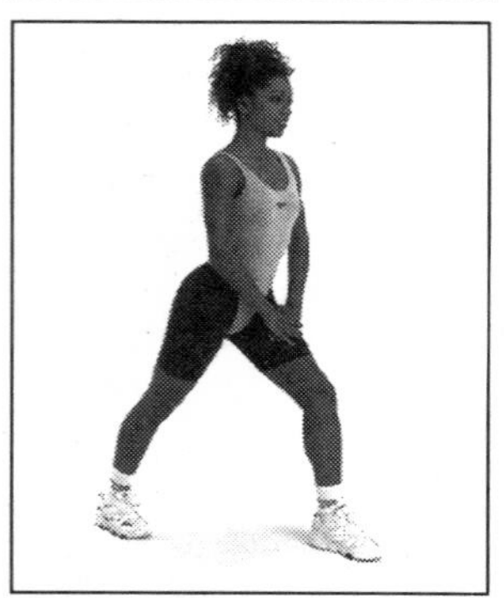

7. Stretch out your shoulders – stand, remembering to keep your posture correct. Bring left arm up and across chest and, using your right hand, gently press left elbow until you feel the stretch. Repeat with right arm.

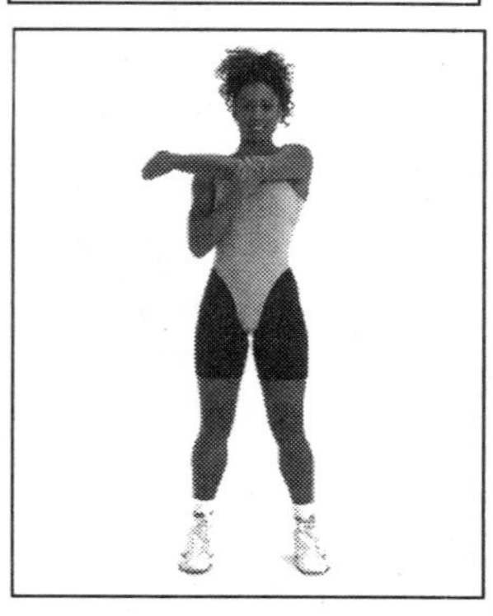

Toning exercises

Repeat each of the following exercises eight times at first, building up to two or three sets of eight with a ten-second pause between each set. Breathe normally throughout, but you will find the exercises easier if you breathe out on the effort and in on the return.

1. Let's start with stomach crunches for a flatter stomach. Lie on your back with knees bent, feet flat on floor, hands placed halfway up thighs. Slowly raise your head and shoulder blades off the floor, using your abdominal muscles to do the work. Gently lower and repeat. To ensure that your neck doesn't do the work, keep a good distance between your chin and your collar bone and keep your neck and shoulders relaxed.

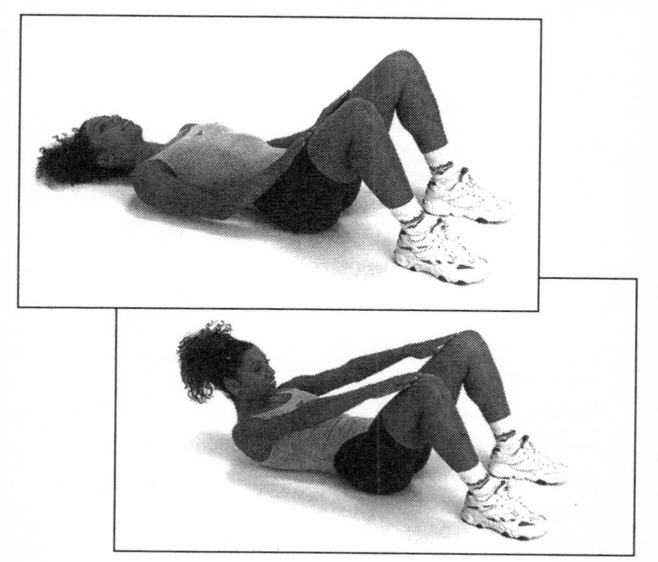

2. To tone your waist, let's move on to diagonal curls. Lie on your back with knees bent, feet flat on floor and hands by your sides. Place your left hand loosely on the right side of your right thigh, halfway up. Keeping your hips flat on floor and your right shoulder pressed into floor, slowly raise your head and left shoulder off the floor and towards your right knee so that your left hand slides beyond right side of right leg. Slowly lower and repeat eight times. Repeat on the other side.

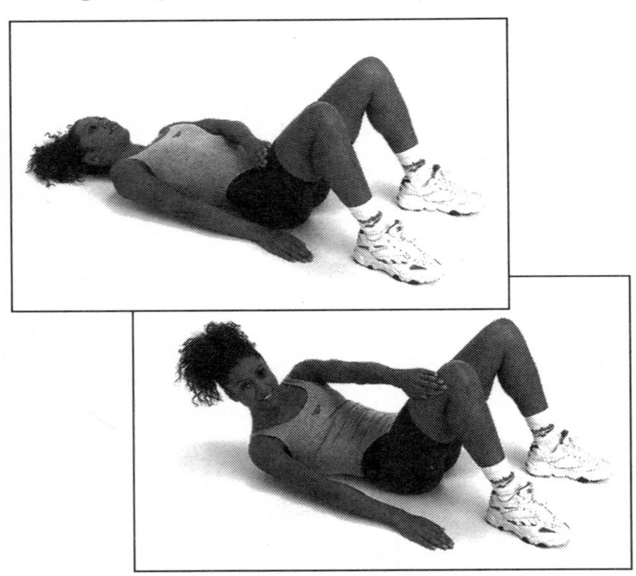

3. Now, let's tone your arms. Grab two full baked bean cans (or use light dumbbells or wrist weights if you have them). Stand with feet hip-width apart, knees relaxed and tummy tucked in. With a can in each hand, start with arms at your sides. Now slowly raise

arms straight up and out to the sides until they are parallel to floor, with the backs of the hands towards the ceiling. Slowly lower and repeat. Now, keeping your back firm and stomach well tucked in, raise your left

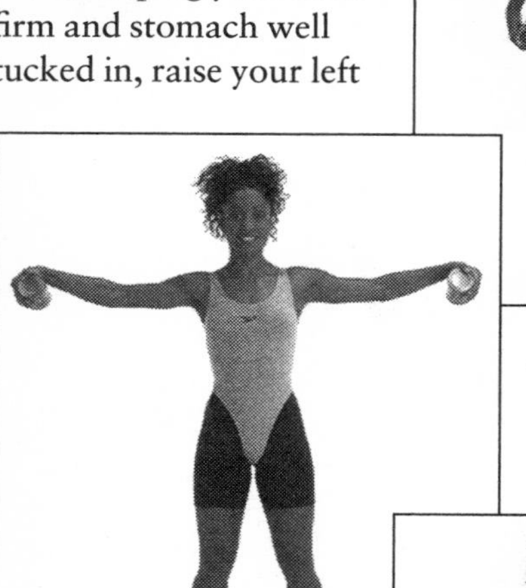

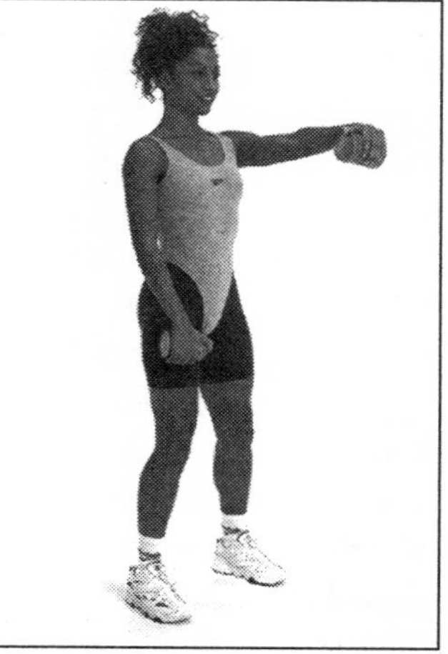

hand straight up in front of you until it is parallel with floor. Hold, and slowly return to the starting position. Repeat with the right arm.

4. More arm toning – your biceps this time. Still standing with feet hip-width apart and holding the cans of beans or weights, fix your elbows into either side of your waist and bring your hands (and weights) up, with palms facing towards body so that left hand/weight touches top of left front shoulder and right hand/weight touches top of right front shoulder. Lower and repeat.

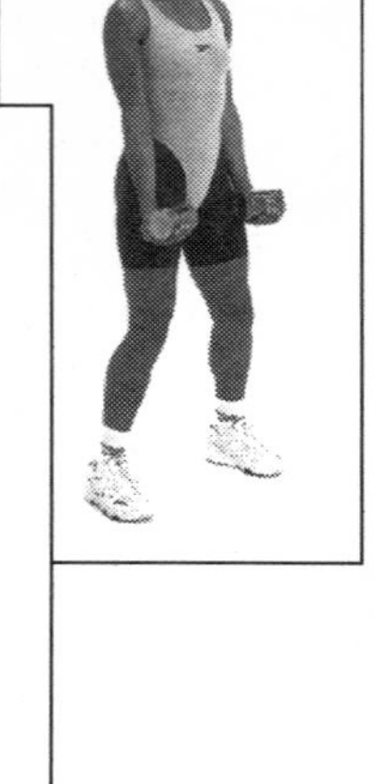

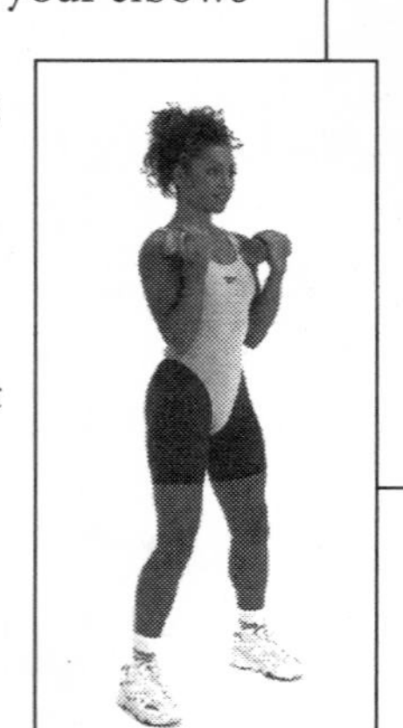

5. Now, let's get your triceps toned. Sit on the floor, knees bent and feet flat on floor, hands on floor to either side of you, fingertips pointing forwards and elbows slightly bent, as shown. Now dip your back down towards the floor, bending your elbows further, as far as is comfortable. Now, using your arms to push

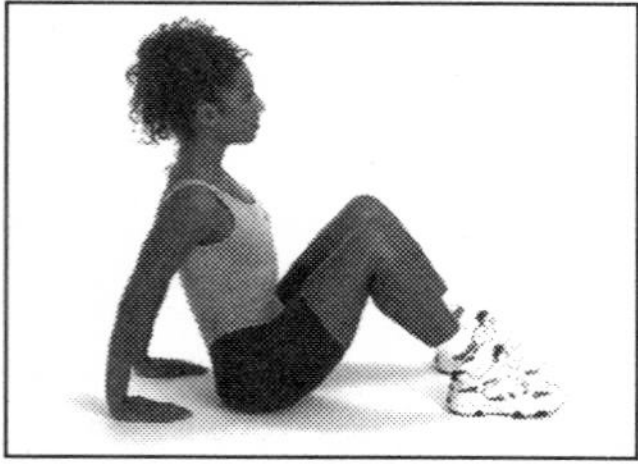

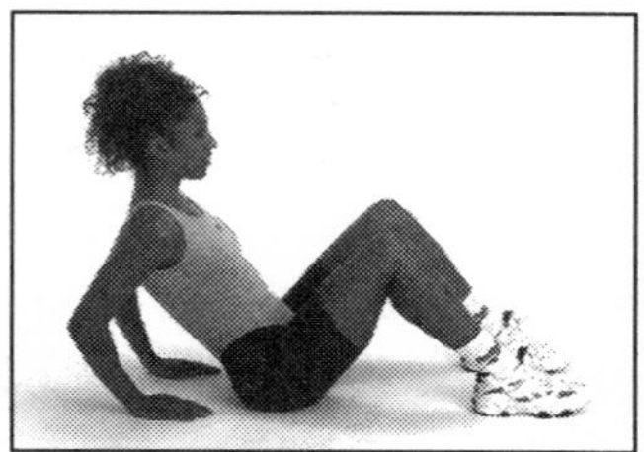

yourself up, slowly raise yourself back to the starting position. Repeat.

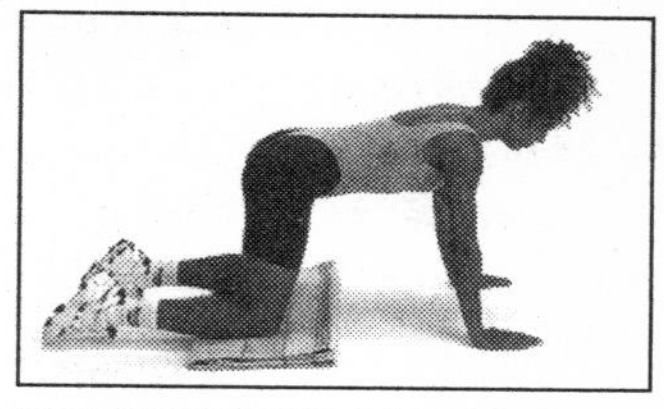

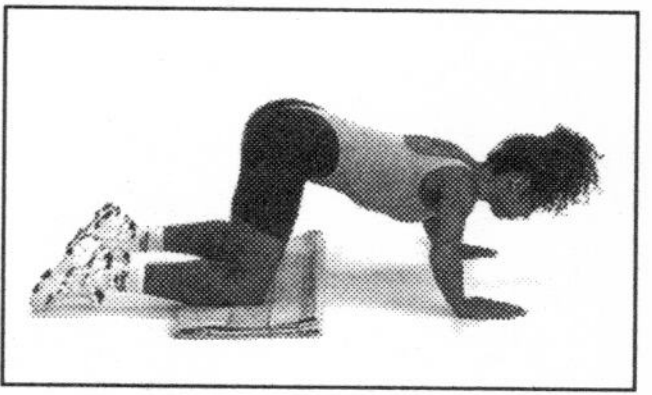

6. For your chest let's do some press-ups. Kneel on all fours with your thighs at right angles to the floor, your back straight and strong and stomach pulled in. Take great care throughout this exercise not to allow the back to arch. Wrists should be in line with your shoulders, and fingers pointing forward. Now slowly lower your chest towards the floor, going as far as you can. Slowly return to the starting position and repeat.

7. Next, we need to work your lower back. Lie on your front with hands clasped loosely behind you and resting on your bottom. Keeping your hips and legs firmly on floor, slowly raise your head and shoulders off floor, squeezing your shoulder blades together. Slowly lower and repeat. Don't flex your neck during this exercise – to prevent this happening, keep looking towards the floor during the exercise.

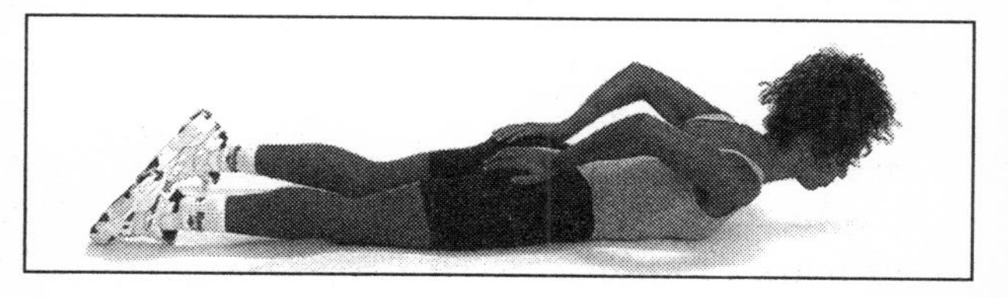

Cool-down stretches

So that your muscles don't ache tomorrow you should take two minutes to do these stretches.

1. *Stomach stretch.* Lie on your front with your head and shoulders off the floor, supported on your arms. Upper arms should be vertical, palms directly in front of your shoulders. Hold this position for a count of sixteen, feeling the stretch along the front of your body.

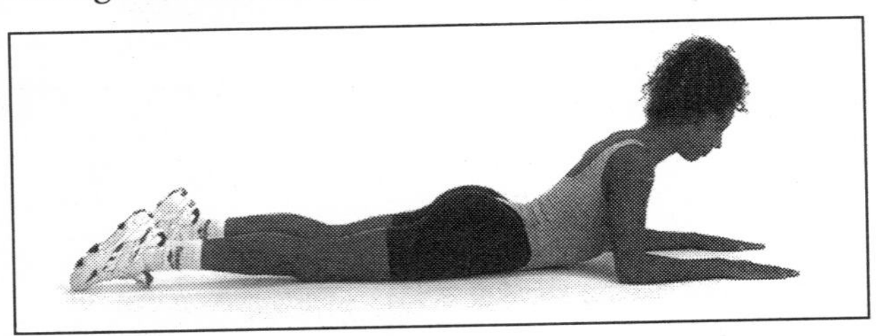

2. *Back stretch.* Kneel on all fours then lower your bottom on to your heels and lower your chest to the floor, keeping your arms stretched out along the floor in front of you, sliding your hands forwards as far as you can. Hold this position for a count of sixteen and feel the stretch all along your back.

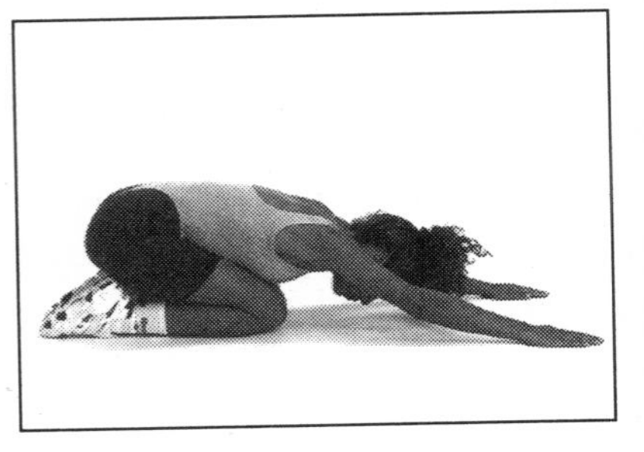

3. *Arm stretch.* Sit on the floor with legs loosely crossed, knees relaxed, tummy tucked in. Raise your right arm up beside your head then bend the elbow and bring the

forearm down behind head so that palm faces inward. Keeping this position, lift your left hand and gently press the right arm just below the elbow so that you achieve a greater stretch. Hold for a count of sixteen. Repeat with the left arm.

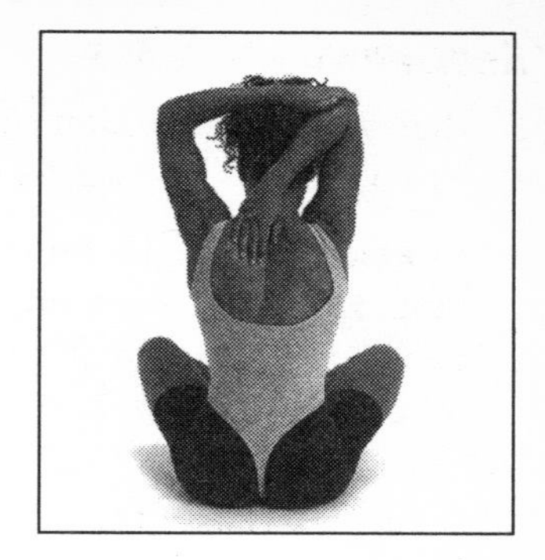

4. ***Waist stretch.*** Sit on the floor with legs crossed. Keeping both hips on the floor, place one hand on the floor to the side of you and reach the other arm up and over. Hold for a count of sixteen, feeling the stretch in your waist. Repeat to the other side.

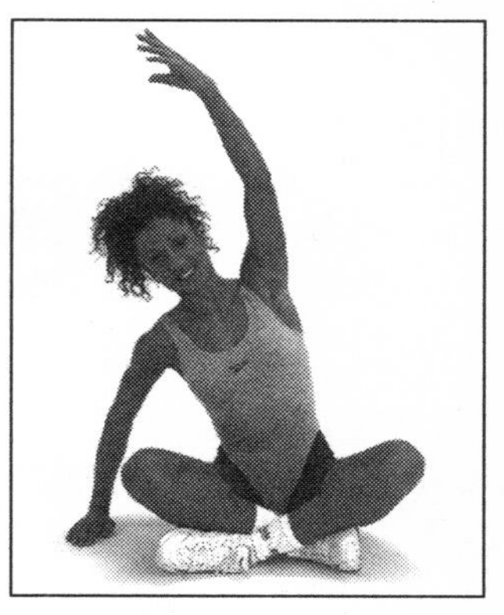

5. ***Hip stretch.*** Still sitting with legs cross, place your hands flat on the floor to either side of one knee. Gently ease forward over that knee, keeping both hips on the floor. Hold for a count of sixteen, feeling the stretch in the opposite hip. Repeat to the other side.

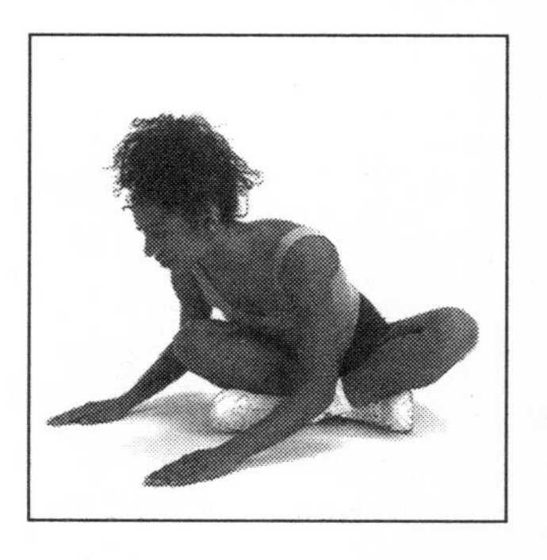

CHAPTER 7

Staying Lean for Life

The *Fat Attack* 30-day plan has, I am sure, shown you that reduced-fat eating can be pleasant, easy and filling. Once you've lost your surplus fat it's not at all difficult to maintain your new, leaner look for the rest of your life.

You'll undoubtedly want to add even more variety to your daily diet and create your own recipes and menus in the weeks, months and years ahead. The guidelines here will ensure that you eat enjoyable but healthy food from now on.

Eat your fill and keep the fat at bay!

As you've seen on the *Fat Attack* plan, it is much more pleasant to lose weight by following a reduced-fat plan than by any other way. A diet with a fat content of 20–25 per cent of total calories allows you to slim without starving.

To maintain your new leaner shape all you need to do is keep the fat calories in your diet to around 25–30 per cent. Again, as with the fat loss plan, the way to do this is to keep a watch on your *saturated* fat intake, keeping it as low as you can.

A *woman* on a average maintenance diet should be getting around 55–65 g of fat a day; a *man* around 70–85 g, of which around 20–25g a day maximum can be saturated (or trans fatty acids) for women and around 25–30g maximum for men.

However, unless you happen to be a nutritionist with a good calculator and plenty of time to spare, there is no way at all you can work out your daily diet in such detail – and there's no real need. If you follow these guidelines you'll be getting the kind of diet that will help to keep you and your heart healthy, and your body lean for good.

Fill up on carbohydrates

As you're reducing your fat intake you'll need to keep eating plenty of the 'complex' carbohydrates – the ones you filled up on while on the 30-day plan. All the following you can safely eat your fill of because they are all high carbohydrate and low fat:

Breads Almost any type of bread except croissants and fried breads, which you should keep for special occasions.

Crispbreads These are fine, and better to eat than lots of cream crackers or traditional cheese biscuits which are relatively high in fat. *Rice cakes* are also good low-fat food and make a nice change.

Potatoes Eat your fill of potatoes, sweet potatoes and roots, baked, boiled or mashed with skimmed milk and a small knob of low-fat spread and seasoning. Roast your potatoes by brushing with olive oil. Check out pages 141–3 for fillings for your baked potatoes.

Rice All types of rice and grains such as couscous, bulgar wheat and pot barley are good for you and filling as well as very versatile. Base more of your meals and recipes around grains. Try quick cook brown rice as a change from white rice – it has a good nutty flavour and keeps you feeling full for ages.

Pasta and Noodles A big plate of steaming pasta with some tangy tomato sauce, or a large bowl of Chinese noodles with a mixed vegetable and turkey stir-fry or one of a thousand other quick and easy recipes – the choice is yours but you should try to fit pasta into your diet at least once or twice a week. Egg pastas contains some fat but not really enough to worry about as part of your healthy diet.

Pulses Pulses are lentils and all the dried beans and peas, almost all of which are now readily available in cans to cut out hours of soaking and cooking time. Baked beans in tomato sauce are fine, but you haven't lived if you haven't tried creamy black-eye beans in a casserole, or lima beans in a salad; brown lentils in a soup or pâté, or chick peas mashed with olive oil and lemon in a pitta.

Not only are pulses very low in fat and high in complex carbohydrate and soluble fibre (the kind that's most beneficial for your heart); they also have an excellent protein, iron and vitamin E content.

Breakfast cereals All of the 'plain' breakfast cereals listed on page 58 are tasty low-fat fillers at any time of day. Muesli contains more fat because of its nut and seed content but even so it is low in saturated fat and high in vitamins and is a much better snack meal than, say, a cream cake!

So all these high-complex-carbohydrate foods are the ones that you'll be filling up on from now on.

Fruit and Vegetables

Fruit and vegetables are also high-carbohydrate foods but much lower in both calories and total carbohydrate content than the foods listed above because they have such a high water content. However, you should continue to eat *plenty* of as wide a variety of fruit and vegetables as you can for the following reasons:

- They help to fill you up
- They fill the plate.
- They contain essential ACE vitamins and other vitamins and minerals.
- They contain fibre.
- They make your diet and recipes versatile and more interesting.
- They look attractive and add colour and pleasure to your diet.

A low intake of fruit and vegetables has been shown time and again to be associated with a higher risk of heart disease and some forms of cancer, so remember – eat up! Even if there are a few kinds you don't like you can *always* find some you do. And don't worry about calorie-counting: almost all fruit and vegetables – except avocados and olives – contain practically no fat. Even those two exceptions contain little saturated fat, so they can be included in your diet without worry.

Get protein in low-fat form

If you're watching your fat intake and eating plenty of carbohydrate the rest of your healthy diet will be made up from lean protein foods. Only about 15 per cent of your total calorie intake needs to be in the form of protein, so most people eat enough without even trying.

The problem can be that many 'protein' foods – such as whole milk, full-fat Cheddar and many cuts of meat – actually contain more *fat* calories than they do *protein* calories. For instance, Cheddar cheese is 25.5 per cent protein but 74.5 per cent fat (and most of that is saturated fat). So you see why it is important to eat mostly the lower-fat protein foods with your carbohydrate, rather than the higher-fat ones.

All the following are low- or reasonably low-fat high-protein foods:

- Chicken and turkey
- Extra lean cooked ham
- Game birds
- Lamb's kidneys
- Rabbit
- Roast beef (lean only)
- Roast pork (lean only)
- Veal
- Venison
- White fish and seafood (oily fish are not low-fat foods but you should still eat plenty of them – see next section)
- Low-fat cottage cheese
- Low-fat fromage frais
- Low-fat yogurt
- Skimmed milk
- Quorn
- Soya mince
- All pulses – dried beans, peas and lentils

If you *mostly* choose from these low-fat protein foods you can, of course, include higher-fat proteins in your diet from time to time.

(*Eggs*, by the way, are quite high in fat and saturated fat and contain a lot of cholesterol – as do *prawns* – and it's best to limit them to 3–4 a week, especially if you are on a low-cholesterol diet on doctor's orders. However, in general, it is more important to limit your intake of saturated fat and to get enough of the 'good for you' fats than it is to worry too much about your cholesterol intake.)

Limit your saturated fat intake

The high-saturated-fat foods are, basically, any animal fats and foods with a high animal fat content – so that means lard, suet, and fatty cuts of meat including the skin of poultry, bacon, fatty ham, and so on. The *lean* cuts of beef, pork and lamb contain only a fraction of the fat of the fatty cuts so you can still enjoy these red meats if you choose the leaner cuts. Duck, also, is not too bad if you simply eat the meat and leave the skin and fat.

Meat products such as luncheon meat, salami, sausages and so on are high in fat (even the low-fat versions of sausages and bacon are quite high in fat so best limited).

Dairy produce – unless included in any of the previous lists – has a high fat content: that means many cheeses, whole milk, butter, eggs, cream and the strained whole-milk yogurts.

Chocolate confectionery is usually high in saturated fat, as are many cakes and biscuits (which often also contain a lot of trans fatty acids).

Pastry products are usually high in saturated fat too (except ready-bought filo). Even pastries made with vegetable oils may be high in the equally bad trans fatty acids.

Fried foods, if they have been cooked in lard or butter, will have quite a high saturated fat content, so it is important to use pure vegetable oils for frying, whenever possible.

Hard margarines, even if made with vegetable oils, are best limited as they are high in trans fatty acids.

These are the foods that you should aim to restrict within your diet, though of course there is no need to give them up altogether. Most of us have foods we can take or leave and if, for instance, you can live without a lot of fatty meat or high-fat cheese or pastry but you really like chocolate – then that's fine. Remember – you are allowed around 10 per cent of the total calories in your diet in the form of saturated fat – so you *do* have some room to include your real favourites.

The thing to remember is to tailor your diet to suit yourself: cut down on the saturated fats that you find easiest to cut down on, and you can have what you do really like in moderation.

Get enough of the 'good for you' fats

As we saw in chapter 1, not all fats are bad for you. While cutting your saturated fat intake down there is no need, in your maintenance diet, to cut down the mono- and polyunsaturated fats. These are the fats that have real positive health benefits (particularly for our hearts and circulatory system) and we should ensure we eat enough of them.

Around 12 per cent of our total diet should be mono-unsaturated fats and around 6 per cent should be poly-unsaturated. Interestingly, our current British diet currently contains roughly the right amounts of these fats, so there is no need to eat *more* of them. But, as we saw in chapter 1, even the high-saturated-fat foods such as meat also contain reasonable amounts of unsaturated fats. By cutting them from our diet we will also be getting less of the unsaturates in these foods – so it's wise to make a conscious effort to take in more mono- and poly-unsaturated fats to make up for this. The best way is to eat more pure vegetable oils, more oily fish and more nuts.

Oils Safflower oil, corn oil, sunflower oil and soya bean oil are highest in the poly-unsaturates, while olive oil, groundnut (peanut) oil and rapeseed oil are highest in the mono-unsaturates.

Because we need slightly more mono-unsaturates in our diet than poly-unsaturates, it is best to get in the habit of using olive, groundnut or rapeseed oil as often as you can. Olive oil does not *all* taste strong and olivy – the more refined types are quite delicate and can be used as well for stir-fries as for salads.

Oily fish Mackerel, herring, salmon, pilchards, sardines, mullet, trout and anchovies are some of the best sources of the fish oils that have been found to help prevent heart disease. As little as two portions a week of these fish can be of benefit. In fact, all fish has a certain amount of these special 'n-3 long chain' fatty acids but these oily fish are much richer sources. So include them in your diet whenever you can.

Fresh nuts Almonds, hazelnuts and peanuts are highest in mono-unsaturates while brazils and walnuts are highest in the poly-unsaturates. Yes – nuts *are* high in calories but a few nuts in their shells make a much healthier TV snack than crisps or chocolate (you'll eat fewer nuts if you have to crack them open than if you buy them ready-shelled!)

Peanut butter is high-calorie but a little goes a long way – try it instead of cheese for a toast topping.

So you see – there is plenty of scope for a delicious and varied diet for you to follow happily for the rest of your long and healthy life.

Remember, you *don't* have to give up every last high-fat treat you enjoy. But if you are like most people who swop to a healthier way of eating and take up some exercise, you'll find your craving for many of your favourites disappears completely in a few weeks.

Fat Attack worked for ...

In just six weeks our four 'guinea pigs' improved their shape, lost inches – and between them shed 59 lb (26.8 kg)!

Eunice Jones **Lost 13 lb (5.9 kg)**

Age: 28 *Height:* 5 ft 3 in (1.6 m)

Starting weight: 10 stone (63.5 kg)
Finishing weight: 9 stone 1 lb (57.6 kg)
Statistics were: 38–29–41 in (97–74–104 cm)
Statistics now: 36–26–38 in (91–66–97 cm)

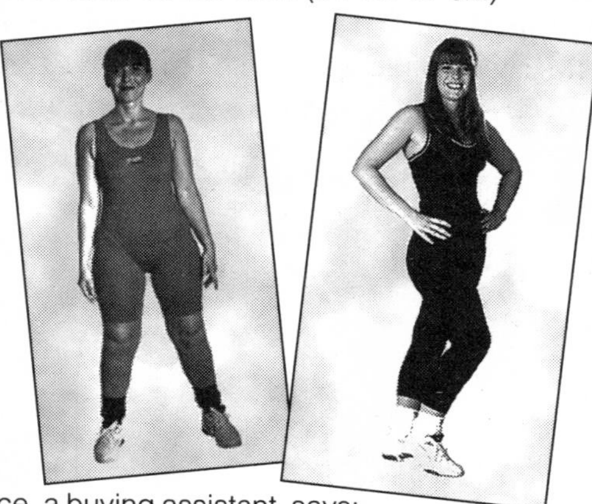

Eunice, a buying assistant, says:

I really enjoyed the workout, and as for the diet – well, I've tried diets before with their weighing and food restrictions, and this just isn't like a diet. It's easy, no fuss – and I can cook meals that look and taste appetising. My friend came round and I cooked her one of the dishes. She said: 'I thought you were supposed to be on a diet!' When I told her I was, she was amazed. It's great. I'll stay with it now to keep my shape.

Jean Shand **Lost 1 stone 1 lb (6.8 kg)**

Age: 28 *Height:* 5 ft 6½ in (1.7 m)

Starting weight: 11 stone 7 lb (73.0 kg)
Finishing weight: 10 stone 6 lb (66.2 kg)
Statistics were: 36–31–38½ in (91–79–98 cm)
Statistics now: 36–29–35 in (91–74–89 cm)

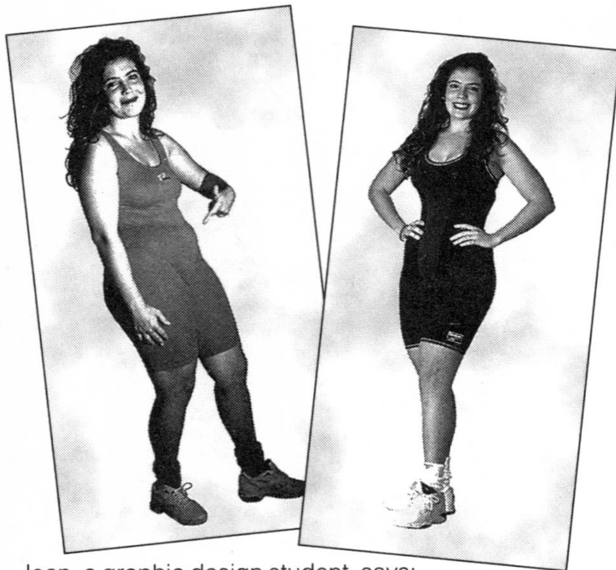

Jean, a graphic design student, says:

I've lost a whole dress size – feeling fitter and looking better gives you so much confidence. I found the workout a bit hard to start with, but I soon began to look forward to doing it. The diet was easy and the portions generous. At first, when sitting down to big platefuls of pasta and potatoes, I thought 'How am I going to shed fat eating all this?' But I did!

Darlene Pickford-Gordon **Lost 13 lb (5.9 kg)**

Age: 34 *Height:* 5 ft 5 in (1.6 m)

Starting weight: 11 stone (69.8 kg)
Finishing weight: 10 stone 1 lb (64.0 kg)
Statistics were: 36–33–44 in (91–84–112 cm)
Statistics now: 35–29–39 in (89–74–99 cm)

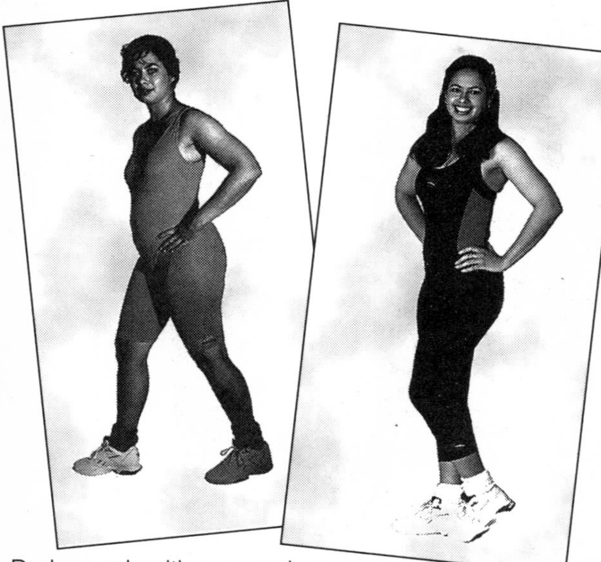

Darlene, a health care worker, says:

I used to feel sluggish with no energy. Now I have tons of energy and do a lot more each day. I swim, walk, dance and feel so much better; I'll never go back to the old days! I enjoyed the Fat Attack plan so much – the workout was inspirational and the diet was tasty, easy and adaptable. It isn't rigid, and it's something you can live with for life – which is what I intend to do!

Gisela Mercati **Lost 1 stone 4 lb (8.2 kg)**

Age: 22 *Height:* 5 ft 7 in (1.7 m)

Starting weight: 14 stone (88.9 kg)
Finishing weight: 12 stone 10lb (80.7 kg)
Statistics were: 38–32–43 in (97–81–109 cm)
Statistics now: 36–28–40 in (91–71–102 cm)

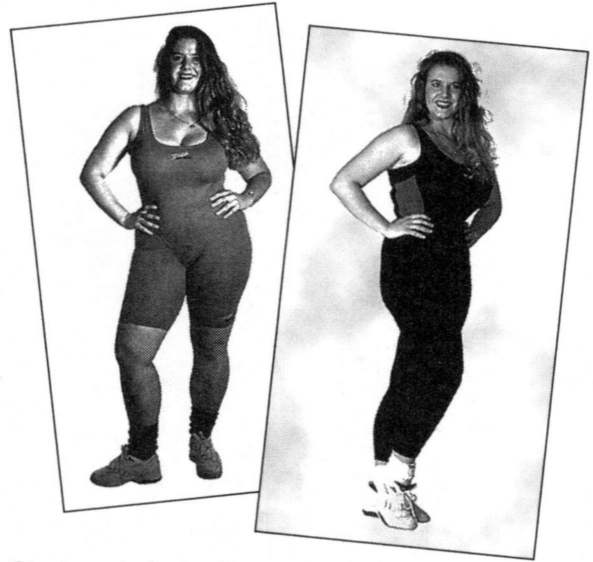

Gisela, a student actress, says:

I'm thrilled with the way I'm shaping up. I would still like to lose another stone or so, but I'm confident I'll do it, because Fat Attack is such a good plan to follow. In my business it's important to have lots of confidence in yourself – and since I'd put on so much weight, that confidence had gone. Now I'm going for it again, and I feel great.